THE COMPA

Series Editor: Y

Compact Clinical Guide to
CHRONIC PAIN MANAGEMENT:
An Evidence-Based Approach for Nurses
Yvonne D'Arcy, MS, CRNP, CNS

Compact Clinical Guide to
ACUTE PAIN MANAGEMENT:
An Evidence-Based Approach for Nurses
Yvonne D'Arcy, MS, CRNP, CNS

Compact Clinical Guide to
CRITICAL CARE, TRAUMA AND EMERGENCY PAIN MANAGEMENT:
An Evidence-Based Approach for Nurses
Liza Marmo, MSN, RN, CCRN

Compact Clinical Guide to
GERIATRIC PAIN MANAGEMENT:
An Evidence-Based Approach for Nurses
Ann Quinlan-Colwell, PhD, RNC, AHNBC, FAAPM

Compact Clinical Guide to
INFANT AND CHILD PAIN MANAGEMENT:
An Evidence-Based Approach for Nurses
Linda L. Oakes, MSN, RN-BC, CCNS

Yvonne D'Arcy, MS, CRNP, CNS, is an expert pain management and palliative care nurse practitioner who has received several awards for nursing excellence, and who possesses a remarkable publishing and presentation career history. Currently, Ms. D'Arcy is the nurse practitioner for pain management and palliative care at Suburban Hospital–Johns Hopkins Medicine, in Bethesda, Maryland. She has significant experience in pain management, having worked as Oncology Pain Service and Staff Education Coordinator at Johns Hopkins Oncology Center; Acute Pain Service Coordinator and Pain Clinic Supervisor at the Mayo Clinic in Jacksonville, Florida; and Pain Center Manager and Clinical Coordinator of the Acute Pain Service at the Heartland Health System in St. Joseph, Missouri. Her accomplishments include delivering more than 100 poster and oral presentations; publishing more than 100 journal articles on pain-related topics; authoring 3 books on pain; and serving on the editorial boards of *Nursing*, *The Journal for Nurse Practitioners*, and *Pain Management News*. Ms. D'Arcy has been an active member of the American Pain Society (where she serves on the guidelines committee), the American Academy of Nurse Practitioners, and the American Society of Pain Management Nurses, having served on various committees and task forces and in executive positions. She is the recipient of the Nursing Spectrum Excellence Award for Advancing and Leading the Profession in the Maryland, Virginia, and Washington, DC, area district and has been awarded a Book of the Year Award by the *American Journal of Nursing* for her book on treating pain in the elderly.

Compact Clinical Guide to

ACUTE PAIN MANAGEMENT

An Evidence-Based Approach for Nurses

Yvonne D'Arcy, MS, CRNP, CNS

SPRINGER PUBLISHING COMPANY
NEW YORK

Springer Publishing Company, LLC
11 West 42nd Street
New York, NY 10036
www.springerpub.com

Acquisitions Editor: Margaret Zuccarini
Senior Editor: Rose Mary Piscitelli
Cover design: Steven Pisano
Composition: Absolute Service, Inc./Pablo Apostol, Project Manager

ISBN: 978-0-8261-0549-3
E-book ISBN: 978-0-8261-0550-9

11 12 13 14 5 4 3 2 1

Library of Congress Cataloging-in-Publication Data
D'Arcy, Yvonne (Yvonne M.), 1946- author.
Compact clinical guide to acute pain management : an evidence-based approach / Yvonne D'Arcy, MS, CRNP, CNS.
p. ; cm. — (Compact clinical guide series)
Includes bibliographical references and index.
ISBN 978-0-8261-0549-3— ISBN 978-0-8261-0550-9 (e-book)
1. Pain—Treatment. 2. Analgesia. I. Title. II. Series: Compact clinical guide series.
[DNLM: 1. Pain—drug therapy. 2. Acute Disease—therapy. 3. Analgesics—therapeutic use. 4. Evidence-Based Medicine. WL 704]
RB127.D3775 2011
616'.0472—dc22

2010050800

Printed in the United States of America by Hamilton Printing

I dedicate this book to my children,
Rob, Lauren, and Leslee, who were an early part of my becoming a nurse and creating my practice as a pain management specialist.

Contents

Preface

I was a nontraditional student when I returned to school for my BSN. I often wondered if I was making the right choice, but after finding myself after graduation on a large medical-surgical unit, I knew that I was always meant to be a nurse. I loved absolutely everything about being a nurse.

After an orthopedic trauma of my own for which I had multiple surgeries and many difficulties with pain management, I went looking for answers to questions about why my pain control had been so poor. As a med-surg nurse, I always felt I did a good job of treating pain in my patients. After my own experiences, I realized that I had missed a lot in treating my patients' pain. I had a new mission: to improve pain management for hospitalized patients, not only for those patients I cared for but for all patients who had pain. I realized that perhaps I was meant to help teach nurses how to better manage pain in their patients by drawing on my own experiences.

As part of my master's program, I developed an acute pain resource nurse program in 1995. The curriculum covered all aspects of acute pain. It was a start to educating nurses in acute pain management, but the program reached only a select few nurses who attended the program.

This book in the Compact Clinical Guide series is aimed at reaching large numbers of practitioners who see many patients who are having all types of acute pain. It provides some basic concepts such as pain transmission and pain medications, and then some specific pain types such as sickle cell and abdominal pain. There are short case studies at the end of each chapter that help to illustrate the concepts of the chapter. All of the information in the book relies heavily on national guidelines and evidence-based materials.

I have worked on several acute pain services over the last 15 years. I hope that by sharing my experience with patients who have acute pain, you will be better able to meet the needs of your own patients with acute pain. I have tried to provide the type of clinical guide that I would have liked to have when I first started my practice. I wish you great success with managing pain in your patients and I hope you will find this guide a useful resource.

Yvonne D'Arcy, MS, CRNP, CNS
Pain Management & Palliative Care Nurse Practitioner
Suburban Hospital–Johns Hopkins Medicine
Bethesda, MD

I

Overview of Acute Pain

1

The Problem of Acute Pain

OVERVIEW OF ACUTE PAIN

The problem of pain is universal. There are relatively few people who have never experienced pain. Those who lack the ability to feel pain because of genetic defects are rare. Most people identify pain as a negative experience and look for a quick way to relieve the pain. In the United States, medicine chests are filled with home remedies and over-the-counter pain relievers. Advertisers supply the American public with examples of products to treat minor sprains, strains, headaches, and muscle aches on television and over the Internet.

Many patients will try to self-treat acute pain that is minor. For more severe unrelieved acute pain needs, patients seek help from health care providers at some type of clinic, emergency room, or hospital.

For all types of health care providers (e.g., nurses, physicians, physical therapists, and pharmacists), the need to know how to assess acute pain, choose an effective treatment, and provide information on effective pain management is critical. Usually, the treatment of mild level acute pain involves some type of medication to relieve pain combined with cold packs, wraps, casts, or slings. For more severe level acute pain from trauma or surgery, more complex techniques are needed, such as intravenous pain medications, patient-controlled analgesia (PCA) or epidural analgesia, or regional analgesic methods, such as nerve blocks using local anesthetics. No matter what type of acute pain a patient has, effective treatment will help ease the pain, decrease the patient's anxiety about getting good pain relief, and decrease the potential for having the pain develop into a chronic or persistent pain condition that is harder to treat.

PREVALENCE OF ACUTE PAIN

It is difficult to determine just what the prevalence of acute pain is because it can be treated in many different places, and it can be the result of many different conditions. From the data that we do have, we know that the prevalence of acute pain is high and that pain can come from various different sources. Whether acute pain is the result of trauma, surgery, or injury, the patient will need to cope with the pain until it resolves after healing takes place. During that time, the patient can experience effects on his or her lifestyle that may limit activity, require analgesic use, and require a period of rehabilitation. Emotional responses to undertreated pain, such as anxiety or fear of pain, can also complicate pain relief and cause the pain to be perceived as more intense, as having a negative impact on function, and as being more invasive into personal lives.

One estimation of the prevalence of acute postoperative pain is based on the finding that out of the 73 million surgeries that took place in 2003, approximately 80% of patients experienced postoperative pain and that 86% of them reported experiencing pain that was either moderate, severe, or extreme (Apfelbaum, Chen, Mehta, & Tong, 2003). Prior to surgery, 59% of these patients indicated that postoperative pain was a concern (Apfelbaum et al., 2003). Consider that 70% of all current surgeries are performed in ambulatory care centers, where quick and effective pain management is a necessity (Apfelbaum et al., 2003). The use of new techniques, adequate medications, and appropriate assessment of medication efficacy for each patient is essential to providing the type of pain relief that patients seek following surgery.

In emergency departments, acute pain is a common complaint. In a midwestern hospital emergency department, a chart review for 1,665 visits during a 7-day period revealed that 61% of patient charts had pain documented in some area of the chart (Cordell et al., 2002). In 52% of the pain charts, pain was documented as the chief complaint (Cordell et al., 2002). In these cases where the patient is seen for a very brief period of time, efficient and effective pain management is a must. Emergency department (ED) care providers of all types need to understand medications for pain, pain assessment, and patient education about pain management. Making effective use of the short time period during which patients are seen in the ED will help provide effective pain relief and prevent readmission.

Good pain management is needed for acute care patients because of the short length of stay most patients with acute pain experience. This is the basis for using the best pain regimen prior to discharge. Ensuring that patients understand how to take medication for pain can help prevent readmission for pain. Readmissions for uncontrolled pain are the most common when compared with all other non pain reasons for readmission in the first week after surgery (Polomano, Dunwoody, Krenzischek, & Rathmell, 2008). The cost of these readmissions totals $1,869 ± $4.553 using mean charges (Coley, Williams, DaPos, Chen, & Smith, 2002). From same-day surgery centers, pain accounts for 36% of all unanticipated admissions and readmissions, with 33% of the patients having had an orthopedic procedure (Coley et al., 2002).

From hospital settings to ED and surgery centers, unrelieved pain is fairly common. Undertreatment can be costly, resulting in readmission for pain treatment or repeated office visits. Nurse practitioners and other health care providers can play an important role in reversing this process by becoming more fully acquainted with appropriate pain assessment tools, learning to use pain medications more effectively, and selecting the appropriate medication for the pain complaint to provide the best opportunity for adequate pain relief.

DIFFERENCES BETWEEN ACUTE AND CHRONIC PAIN

There are considerable differences between acute pain and chronic pain. Differences occur in the time frame for the pain complaint, but perhaps more importantly, in the pathophysiology of the pain and the appropriate choice of treatments that can deliver the most effective relief for that pain. Learning the differences between the types of pain can help the health care provider choose the best methods for treating pain.

Acute Pain

Acute pain is very different from chronic, persistent pain. Acute pain usually has a short duration and has an identifiable cause, such as trauma, injury, or surgery (American Pain Society [APS], 2008; American Society for Pain Management Nursing [ASPMN], 2010). The source of acute pain is tissue damage, and the sensation of pain warns the body that it has been injured. The duration of acute pain is expected by the patient to be short-term and to resolve as the injury heals.

Anxiety is common with acute pain. There may also be some sympathetic nervous system activity, such as increases in heart rate or respiratory rate. Acute pain can also cause diaphoresis, nausea, and vomiting related to the pain, and/or pallor. Once the pain is controlled, the patient can relax and additional signs and symptoms may lessen or resolve.

Clinical Pearl

Do not base your assumption on the presence of pain by observing changes in blood pressure or increased heart rate. These may be caused by other responses, such as anxiety or fear, and may not be a result of the pain. Patients with chronic pain accommodate the continued pain and do not typically experience these physiological changes.

Chronic Pain

Chronic pain, on the other hand, is pain that lasts beyond the normal healing period, which is usually longer than 3 to 6 months (APS, 2008). Chronic pain has no purpose and can exist without visible injury. Some patients with chronic pain can relate a specific incident, such as surgery, a fall, or injury, to the onset of the pain. Other patients just wake up with pain that continues despite all the best efforts at treatment. Chronic pain can also be the result of cancer, related to the spread of the disease, tumor growth, or side effects of chemotherapy. Chronic pain does not need tissue injury to exist, and physical damage may not be evident on X-ray, magnetic resonance imaging (MRI), or computed tomography (CT); nonetheless, the pain persists.

Patients with chronic pain who are experiencing acute pain may have no visible response to the new pain. Because chronic pain is a daily phenomenon, most patients accommodate to the pain experiences, do not expect to be pain free, and will tolerate high levels of pain on a daily basis. Patients with chronic pain, such as from cancer, will not often demonstrate signs of sympathetic nervous system (SNS) activation, such as increased pulse or heart rate (APS, 2008).

The lack of response to acute pain in patients with chronic, persistent pain can be confusing for health care providers. Many providers expect to see high levels of pain behaviors, such as guarding, moaning, crying, or withdrawing, from patients when the pain is rated as severe. However, for the patient with chronic pain who is experiencing acute pain, there may be few, if any, indications of the pain, let alone any outward signs consistent with high levels of pain. For patients with chronic pain who are experiencing acute pain, the same type of pain assessment is performed in which the patient is asked to rate the pain using the Numeric Rating Scale (NRS)—the 11-point Likert scale from 0 to 10—where 0 is no pain and 10 is the worst pain imaginable. The number is then used to choose an intervention to treat the pain complaint. More information on assessing pain and on acute pain in patients with chronic pain will be provided in later chapters of the book.

One very important aspect of treating acute pain is the concept that untreated or undertreated acute pain can progress to a chronic pain condition that is much more difficult to treat (APS, 2008; Macintyre, Scott, Schug, Visser, & Walker, 2005). One perfect example of this is complex regional pain syndrome (CRPS), formerly called reflex sympathetic dystrophy syndrome (RSDS).

Patients who are candidates for the development of CRPS include the following:

- Patients with surgical nerve injury or trauma.
- Patients with crush-type injuries with prolonged, persistent pain.
- Patients who report high levels of unrelieved pain after acute injury or surgery, despite changes in treatment.

As pain stimuli continuously present to peripheral neurons in a constant feedback loop, the pain experienced can be converted to a centrally controlled pain condition, such as CRPS, that is difficult to treat and is less responsive to ordinary pain medications. There are two types of CRPS: *Type I*, which corresponds to the older RSDS category and occurs without a nerve lesion; and *Type II*, which was formerly called causalgia, and has a detectable nerve lesion (Rowbotham, 1998).

For a pain condition to be diagnosed as CRPS, some of the following criteria must be present:

- Regional pain—usually in the upper or lower extremities
- Sensory motor changes—sudomotor abnormalities
- Changes to the skin
- Thickening of the nails
- Hair loss in the affected area

Although CRPS is considered to be a chronic condition, it can develop in acute care patients as they undergo repeated surgeries, frequent débridements, or other types of procedures that cause continuous injury to tissue or nerves at the same site. Some of the telltale complaints of patients with developing CRPS include the sensation of burning pain; painful numbness; sensitivity to temperature changes, cold especially; and pain out of proportion to the injury. The recommendation from pain management specialists is to treat acute pain aggressively to limit the effect on the individual and to decrease the potential for the development of CRPS (D'Arcy, 2007; Macintyre et al., 2005).

The acute care nurse practitioner learning to identify the signs and symptoms of developing neuropathic pain such as CRPS can make an immeasurable difference to the final outcome for the patient. If the condition is identified and aggressive pain management occurs quickly, the chance that the pain can be minimized and treated effectively is dramatically increased. Use of medications designed for treating neuropathic pain, such as antiepileptic medications or antidepressants, make the difference in being able to return to a normal lifestyle after the injury or surgery as opposed to dealing with a chronic pain condition for the remainder of the patient's life.

Neuropathic Pain

CRPS is just one type of pain that is called neuropathic pain—pain that is caused by an injury to a peripheral nerve or the central nervous system, or CNS (ASPMN, 2010; Staats et al., 2004). Neuropathic pain is a type of chronic pain, but it may have its source in an acute pain condition. Some of the causes of neuropathic pain include the following:

- Nerve damage from surgery, such as an entrapment syndrome, postthoracotomy pain, postmastectomy pain syndrome, phantom limb or breast pain, or posthysterectomy pain
- Neuropathy from a disease or injury, such as postherpetic neuralgia, diabetes, or CRPS
- Neuropathic pain as the result of treatments, such as chemotherapy, especially when using such agents as vinca alkaloid or other chemotherapeutic agents
- Centrally originating pain syndromes, such as poststroke pain, fibromyalgia, and spinal cord injury pain (List taken from Berry, Covington, Dahl, Katz, & Miaskowski, 2006; D'Arcy, 2007)

Although some acute pain conditions may lead to chronic pain syndrome, if the condition has a neuropathic component, it is by far more difficult to treat, and the suffering the patient endures is much more destructive to a patient's quality of life, is more intense, and is long term. The key to differentiating neuropathic pain from a less complex chronic pain is the use of descriptors such as burning, painful tingling, or numbness. More information on neuropathic pain descriptors will be provided in the chapter on pain assessment.

PAIN TRANSMISSION

Pain Theories

Some of the mechanisms of pain transmission are different for acute pain and chronic pain (Figure 1.1). The onset of acute pain is sudden and can provoke a fight or flight type of response, with adrenaline release that will subside rapidly. On the other hand, chronic pain is long term and can become more complex over time, and advanced pain facilitating responses such as the activation of *N*-methyl-d-aspartic acid (NMDA) receptors takes place. Many pharmaceutical companies aim the action of their medications at a specific site in the pain transmission process. For example, interfering with serotonin at the synaptic junction can help reduce the amount of pain-facilitating substances available to create or continue the pain stimulus.

There are multiple theories advanced over the years about how pain is transmitted and what physiologic mechanisms are involved. One of the earliest theorists was René Descartes, who felt that pain was a stimulus–response mechanism. This concept was also called the labeled line theory (Cervero, 2005). Using this theory, pain was seen as a painful stimulus that traveled up to the brain, resulting in the body recognizing the sensation as pain. An example is a pain stimulus caused by a burn or trauma that travels from the site of the burn or trauma to the brain, where the brain recognizes the stimulus as pain. The resulting response would be for the body to withdraw from the source of pain (e.g., removing the hand from a fire or otherwise pulling the affected area away from the source of the pain). This theory focuses primarily on the physical aspect of pain rather than including the emotional or psychological aspects of the pain experience.

Especially for patients with chronic pain, the psychologic and emotional component of pain is an important aspect of the condition. Older theories, such as those espoused by Pavlov, considered

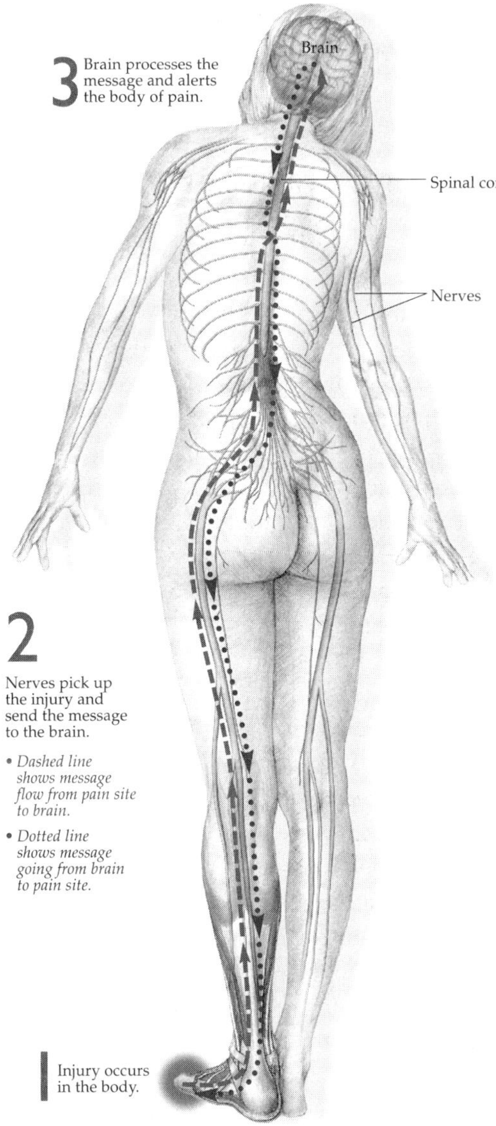

Brain
3 Brain processes the message and alerts the body of pain.
Spinal cord
Nerves
2
Nerves pick up the injury and send the message to the brain.
• Dashed line shows message flow from pain site to brain.
• Dotted line shows message going from brain to pain site.
1 Injury occurs in the body.

Figure 1.1 ■ Pain transmission—Exemplar. *Source:* Used by permission of Anatomical Charts, Park Ridge, IL.

pain to be a learned response that was affected by cultural and learned behaviors that could be offset by operant conditioning (Fordyce, 1976; Pavlov, 1927). A contemporary theorist, Turk, described pain as a multidimensional experience and proposed that the patient, not the health care practitioner, is the specialist on his or her pain (Turk, 2003). This theory empowers patients to become an active participant in pain treatment and helps patients to diminish negative behaviors and increase positive reinforcing behaviors (ASPMN, 2010).

Perhaps the most well-known theory of pain transmission is the gate control theory developed by Melzack and Wall in 1965 (ASPMN, 2010). In this theory, the psychological and physiologic aspects of pain transmission are combined. Quite simply, the gate control theory states that a pain stimulus can be of significant intensity to "open" a neuronal gate, allowing the pain stimulus to proceed through the nervous system to the brain to create a sensation that can be identified as pain.

The actual steps in pain transmission using the gate control theory include the following:

- A pain stimulus from the body periphery is carried by A delta and C nerve fibers to the dorsal horn of the spinal cord.
- The gate is located in the substantia gelatinosa in the dorsal horn of the spinal cord and it can facilitate or inhibit (either promote or stop) the progression of the nerve impulse through the CNS.
- If the painful stimulus is of sufficient intensity or persists, the pain is transmitted up through the limbic system to the cerebral cortex.
- In the cerebral cortex, the stimulus is recognized as pain and the efferent neural path is activated to provide a response to the pain (Adapted from ASPMN, 2010).

As science has investigated and furthered the knowledge of this pain transmission theory, several other concepts have emerged. These include the following:

- The central control processes and central intensity processes located in the brain and limbic system help to translate the understanding of the sensation and can modulate the section of the descending pain pathways.

- When pain stimuli entering the nervous system reaches critical levels, the T-cell system is activated, which creates a link between the brain and the body to link the subjective and objective experience of pain.
- By increasing the sensation of pain, peripheral nerve sensitization can be caused through continued nerve stimulation, producing a state of *hyperexcitability* because of alternation in the sodium ion channels. Continued pain stimulation can be increased as the inflammatory response persists.
- *Wind up* and *neuroplasticity* can also occur. Wind up is a phenomenon that develops when, as the result of continued moderate-to-severe pain, the NMDA receptors are activated. These receptors serve to process the pain faster and with more intensity, creating pain intensity that is greater than expected for the stimulus. The pain response is greatly enhanced when wind up has occurred. *Central sensitization* can occur as a result of wind up, which allows normal tissue to become extremely sensitive to pressure in areas that are not identified as painful. Neuroplasticity is the result of a moderate-to-severe pain that lasts for more than 24 hours and occurs in the spinal area of the nervous system. With neuroplasticity, pain fiber growth is stimulated and the pain inhibition system is damaged, resulting in more intense pain that is widespread and lessening the ability of the body to stop pain. *Peripheral sensitization* can occur as a result of neuroplasticity. This condition creates another condition in which nonpainful touch and pressure become painful (ASPMN, 2010; Berry et al., 2006; Yaksh, 2005).

As we study and begin to understand the process and theory of pain transmission, more information about the process is discovered. As science expands its understanding of the pathophysiology of pain, more information will lead to a better understanding of the transmission process.

The Concept of Nociception

How is pain really felt? The concept of nociception can help to determine just how pain moves through the nervous system, and it can also provide us with ideas about interference with pain facilitation and inhibition. *Nociception* is defined as the perception of pain by sensory pain receptors called *nociceptors* located in the periphery (Sorkin, 2005). The theory of nociception suggests that there are four stages, or levels, of pain transmission.

Stage 1. *Transduction*—A noxious stimuli converts energy into a nerve impulse, which is detected by sensory receptors called nociceptors.
Stage 2. *Transmission*—The neural pain signal moves from the periphery to the spinal cord and brain.
Stage 3. *Perception*—The pain impulse is transmitted to the higher areas of the brain, where it is identified as pain.
Stage 4. *Modulation*—Facilitation and inhibitory input form the brain modulates or influences the sensory transmission at the level of the spinal cord (Berry et al., 2006; D'Arcy, 2007).

The transmission of pain is the passing along of a pain stimulus from the peripheral nervous system (PNS) into the CNS, where it is translated and recognized as pain. The afferent nerve fibers move the stimulus along the neuronal pathways.

Nociception can come from various locations: *visceral*, where pain is identified as crampy or gnawing pain; or *somatic*, pain from skin, muscles, bones, and joints identified by patients as sharp pain (Berry et al., 2006). The following are several different types of receptors that can trigger a pain response:

- *Mechanoreceptors*—activated by pressure
- *Thermal receptors*—activated by heat or cold
- *Chemoreceptors*—activated by chemicals; for example, inflammatory substances (ASPMN, 2010)

Peripheral Pain Transmission

Pain can first be experienced by free nerve endings or nociceptors located in the periphery of the body. As a person cuts a hand or fractures an extremity, the pain stimulus is first perceived in the nerves closest to the injury. For a pain stimulus to be created, the sodium ions on the nerve fiber must depolarize, which causes the pain stimulus to be produced and passed along the neural circuitry.

The following are two main types of nerves that transmit pain impulses or stimuli:

- *A-delta fibers* are large nerve fibers covered in myelin that can transmit a nerve impulse rapidly. The pain transmitted on an A-delta fiber is easily localized, and the patients may describe the pain as sharp or stabbing.
- *C fibers* are smaller and unmyelinated, and the pain impulse is conducted at a much slower rate. Pain that is produced by C fibers is identified by patients as achy or burning (ASPMN, 2010; Sorkin, 2005).

Two primary substances can help facilitate the transmission of pain from the periphery. *Substance P* is a neurotransmitter secreted by the free nerve endings of C fibers, the function of which is to speed the transmission of the pain impulse. *Bradykinin* is a second type of neurotransmitter, the function of which is to participate in the inflammatory response and hyperalgesia (ASPMN, 2010). Nociception can stimulate both A-delta and C fibers for pain transmission.

Other substances that participate in the facilitation of pain include the following:

- *Histamine* is a substance released from mast cells produced in response to tissue trauma.
- *Serotonin* can be released from platelets and is produced in response to tissue trauma.
- *COX products (prostaglandin E_2 and thromboxane E_2)* act to sensitize and excite C fibers, causing hyperexcitability.
- *Cytokines* (*interleukins and tumor necrosis factor* [TNF]) can sensitize C fiber terminals and participate in the inflammatory and infection process involving mast cells.
- *Calcitonin gene-related peptide* (CGRP) is located at C fiber nerve endings and produces local cutaneous vasodilatation, plasma extravasation, and skin sanitization in collaboration with substance P production. (ASPMN, 2010; Berry et al., 2006; Sorkin, 2005)

Once transduction takes place, the nerve impulse is passed through a synaptic junction from the PNS to the CNS. This synaptic junction has various functions and secretes substances. Some medications (e.g., *pregabalin*) act at the synaptic junction by blocking calcium channels. This, in turn, can reduce the amount of neuronal firing and decrease the passage of pain stimuli. The synapse is between the peripheral neuron into the CNS via the dorsal root ganglion.

Central Nervous System Pain Transmission

As the pain stimulus is passed from the PNS into the CNS, the signal passes through the dorsal root ganglion to a synaptic junction in the substantia gelatinosa, located in the dorsal horn of the spinal cord. As the stimulus pushing the pain impulse forward overcomes any opposing or inhibiting forces, the "gate" is opened, allowing the pain impulse to proceed up the spinal cord to the limbic system and brain.

The opening of the gate is controlled by a summing of all the forces involved in the conduction of the pain impulse. If the facilitating forces, neural excitability, and pain-facilitating substances (such as substance P) predominate, the pain impulse is passed on. If pain-inhibiting forces predominate, the signal is blocked and the gate does not open. If, by chance, the pain impulse is perceived as potentially life threatening, a reflex arc across the spinal cord will fire, causing an immediate response to protect the affected area (e.g., touching a hot surface causes the body to retract and remove the hand from the hot surface). This event can take place before any central processing of the neural signal begins (Cervero, 2005).

Centrally active pain-facilitating and pain-inhibiting substances include the following:

Facilitating:

- Substance P
- Glutamate—responsible for the communication between the peripheral and central nervous system (Rowbotham, Kidd, & Porecca, 2006); also plays a role in activating the NMDA receptors (Mersky, Loeser, & Dubner, 2005)
- Aspartate
- Cholecystokinin
- CGRP
- Nitric oxide

Inhibitory:

- Dynorphin—an endogenous opioid
- Enkephalin
- Norepinephrine
- Serotonin
- B-endorphin—an endogenous opioid
- Gamma-aminobutyric acid (GABA) (ASPMN, 2010; Sorkin, 2005)

Also performing an inhibitory role are the opioid receptors located both presynaptically and postsynaptically that are available for binding opioid substances, such as morphine, and producing analgesia. Although there are opioid receptors located at other sites in the body, those that are located inside the spinal cord are the most well understood in how they function.

As the pain impulse passes through the dorsal horn of the *spinal cord*, it passes across the spine to the lateral spinothalamic tracts. The *pain impulse* proceeds up the spinal cord to the thalamus and limbic system. This *activates* the emotions and memories associated with pain, which are then passed to the cerebral cortex where the pain impulse or stimulus is recognized as pain. Although this process seems complicated, the body can transmit a pain impulse in milliseconds.

Two pain substances are active within the limbic system: *norepinephrine* and *serotonin*. Current drug therapies, such as tricyclic antidepressants and selective serotonin reuptake inhibitors (SSRIs), are aimed at reducing the amount of serotonin available to activate neuronal firing at synaptic junctions. The synaptic junctions have various functions. They not only produce pain impulses but also can influence pain by reducing the amount of pain-facilitating substances.

Once the pain stimulus reaches the cerebral cortex, the ascending pathway is completed. Once the pain is identified, the response is passed down along the descending neural pathways to the periphery. The descending impulse uses nerve fibers from the locus coeruleus and periaqueductal gray matter to pass the pain impulse downward so that the response to move the hand away from a hot surface, for example, occurs. The overall pain transmission relies on both the neural pathways and the neurotransmitters.

SUMMARY

Although pain is a very common patient complaint, there are distinct differences between acute and chronic, or persistent, pain. Health care providers treating patients with pain should be able to recognize the differences between pain types and treat the type of pain accordingly. Acute pain may respond to the typical analgesic, whereas chronic pain conditions may require a combined medication and complementary techniques plan of care. Treating acute pain effectively can help prevent the development of a chronic pain condition, such as CRPS, that can be much more difficult to treat.

Understanding how pain is produced in the body can help health care providers learn to identify the way it is expressed physically by patients. Patients will often describe pain as achy or sharp, and knowing that different mechanisms and nerve fibers are producing this presentation can help the provider better identify the source of the pain.

The production of pain is a very sophisticated, complex process that can be difficult to understand. Learning the mechanism of acute pain production and the facilitating and inhibitory substances can help a health care provider understand why medications such as antidepressants and antiepileptic medication can decrease pain. More information on medication mechanisms of action will be provided in the medication chapter.

Case Study

This case study indicates the type of patient scenarios that will be included in each chapter. Some of the information needed to answer the questions in this presentation can be found in the assessment and medication chapters.

Peggy Smith is a 65-year-old patient who was hanging Christmas lights on the front of her home when she fell from the ladder she was on. She landed on her left hip and now has significant pain with an external rotation to her left lower extremity. She was taken to the hospital by an ambulance, where she is diagnosed with a hip fracture and prepared for surgery to correct the deformity.

In the ED, Peggy is complaining of significant pain at 8 out of 10 level. When the triage nurse takes her history, Peggy relates a history of chronic, persistent pain in her low back from a motor vehicle accident that occurred 6 years ago. She takes four oxycodone with acetaminophen tablets every day for her back pain and occasionally receives an epidural steroid injection for a radicular pain that goes down her left leg. She drinks a glass of wine every day at dinner and occasionally will have alcohol when she is out with friends. How will you treat Peggy's pain?

Questions to Consider

1. Does the fact that Peggy has chronic pain affect her new acute pain?
2. Because Peggy takes opioid medication every day, will her pain medication needs be different? If so, how will you adjust the doses of medication to accommodate the acute pain?
3. Is Peggy addicted to her usual pain medications?
4. What role does Peggy's alcohol use play in her management needs?
5. What is the best type of pain management for Peggy in the postoperative time period? Does her age affect your decision?

REFERENCES

American Pain Society. (2008). *Principles of analgesic use in the treatment of acute pain and cancer pain*. Glenview, IL: Author.

American Society for Pain Management Nursing. (2010). *Core curriculum for pain management nursing* (2nd ed.). Dubuque, IA: Kendall Hunt Publishing Company.

Apfelbaum, J., Chen, C., Mehta, S., & Tong, G. (2003). Postoperative pain experience: Results from a national survey suggests postoperative pain continues to be undermanaged. *Anesthesia & Analgesia, 97*(2), 534–540.

Berry, P. H., Covington, E., Dahl, J., Katz, J., & Miaskowski, C. (2006). *Pain: Current understanding of assessment, management, and treatments*. Reston, VA: National Pharmaceutical Council, Inc.

Cervero, F. (2005). The gate control theory, then and now. In H. Mersky, J. Loeser, & R. Dubner (Eds.), *Paths of pain*. Seattle, WA: IASP Press.

Coley, K., Williams, B., DaPos, S., Chen, C., & Smith R. (2002). Retrospective evaluation of unanticipated admissions and readmissions after same day surgery and associated costs. *Journal of Clinical Anesthesia, 14*(5), 349–353.

Cordell, W., Keene, K., Giles, B., Jones, J. B., Jones, J. H., & Brizendine E. (2002). The high prevalence of pain in emergency medical care. *American Journal of Emergency Medicine, 20*(3), 165–169.

D'Arcy, Y. (2007). *Pain management: Evidence-based tools and techniques for nursing professionals.* Marblehead, MA: HCPro, Inc.

Fordyce, W. E. (1976). *Behavioral methods for chronic pain and illness.* St. Louis, MO: C. V. Mosby.

Macintyre, P. E., Scott, D. A., Schug, S. A., Visser, E. J., & Walker, S. M. (2005). *Acute pain management: Scientific evidence* (2nd ed.). Melbourne, Australia: Australian and New Zealand College of Anaesthetists and Faculty of Pain Medicine.

Melzack, R., & Wall, P. (1965). Pain mechanisms: A new theory. *Science, 150*(699), 971–979.

Mersky, H., Loeser, J. D., & Dubner, R. (2005). *The paths of pain: 1975–2005.* Seattle, WA: IASP Press.

Pavlov, I. P. (1927). *Conditioned reflexes.* Oxford, England: Humphrey Milford.

Polomano, R., Dunwoody, C., Krenzischek, D., & Rathmell, J. (2008). *Pain Management Nursing, 9*(1), S3–S10.

Rowbotham, M. C. (1998). Complex regional pain syndrome type I (reflex sympathetic dystrophy): More than a myth. *Neurology, 51*(1), 4–5.

Rowbotham, M. C., Kidd, B. L., & Porreca, F. (2006). Role of central sensitization in chronic pain: Osteoarthritis and rheumatoid arthritis compared to neuropathic pain. In H. Flor, E. Kalso, & J. Dostrovsky (Eds.), *Proceedings of the 11th World Congress on Pain* (pp. 231–249). Seattle, WA: IASP Press.

Sorkin, L. (2005). Nociceptive pain. In M. S. Wallace & P. S. Staats (Eds.), *Pain medicine & management.* New York: McGraw-Hill.

Staats, P., Argoff, C., Brewer, R., D'Arcy, Y., Gallagher, R., McCarberg, B., Reisner, L. (2004). Neuropathic pain: Incorporating new consensus guidelines into the reality of clinical practice. *Advanced Studies in Medicine, 4*(7B), S542–582.

Turk, D. (2003). Cognitive behavioral approach to the treatment of chronic pain patients. *Regional Anesthesia and Pain Medicine, 28*(6), 573–579.

Yaksh, T. (2005). Neuropathic pain. In M. S. Wallace & P. S. Staats (Eds.), *Pain medicine & management.* New York: McGraw-Hill.

2

Standards, Guidelines, Practice Statements, and The Joint Commission Standard for Acute Pain Management

OVERVIEW

The awareness of the problem of undertreated acute pain has existed since the 1973, when Marks and Sachar discovered that residents and physicians did not understand how to treat acute pain and that patients reported high levels of pain that were untreated or undertreated. Since that time, much effort and many interventions were aimed at increasing the quality of pain management for acute care patients. Congress created the *Decade of Pain from 2000 to 2010,* focusing on how to improve pain management; however, not much has changed. Many patients still report undertreated pain and, as a result, more formalized standards have been developed by The Joint Commission to guide the practice of pain management in centers that are accredited by The Joint Commission.

From the patient perspective, there is an increasing awareness that people are entitled to adequate pain relief. Using the Internet and printed media, patients have been able to access hospital ratings for service and provision of pain management. They understand that pain management can be achieved with various medications and techniques. Many patients refer to their pain using the numeric 0 to 10 pain intensity scale without needing a prompt from the health care provider. Most hospitals have a patient bill of rights that outlines what patients can expect from the hospital, including the right to have their pain assessed, reassessed regularly, and adequately treated.

For health care providers working in acute care, knowing what The Joint Commission requires and what national guidelines recommend as appropriate care provides a basis for practice. More importantly, knowing how to manage the patient's pain because it is the right thing to do for the patient is really the guiding principle of care.

National Guidelines for Treating Pain

There are more than 500 guidelines for acute pain listed in the national guideline database at the Guideline Clearinghouse (www.guideline.gov). Most of the guidelines apply to a specific type of acute pain, such as, for example, pain with myocardial infarction, postoperative pain, or orthopedic injury pain.

National societies and organizations draft position papers and guidelines for the treatment of certain pain conditions or pain at certain times during treatment. Guidelines related to treating pain can be found at the following sites:

- American Pain Society (APS)—www.ampainsoc.org: Low back pain, cancer pain, fibromyalgia pain, acute pain, chronic opioid therapy (COT), pain management in primary care
- American Society of Anesthesiologists—www.asahq.org: Perioperative guideline
- American Pain Foundation—www.painfoundation.org: Help for finding general pain information
- American Academy of Pain Medicine—www.painmed.org: Position statements on practice issues
- American Society for Pain Management Nursing—www.aspmn.org: Position statements
- American Society for PeriAnesthesia Nursing—www.aspan.org: Pain and comfort and postoperative nausea guidelines
- Oncology Nursing Society—www.ons.org: Cancer pain management information
- American Society of Regional Anesthesia (ASRA)—www.asra.com: Epidural/Anticoagulation position statement
- American Geriatrics Society—www.americangeriatrics.org: Guidelines and statement on pain in older patients Veterans Affairs/Department

of Defense (VA/DOD) guidelines for pain management available at www.healthquality.va.gov.

These are only a sampling of pain-related guidelines and position papers that can be used to find current, evidence-based information about pain management. More websites and disease-specific websites, such as the fibromyalgia website, can offer additional information on the current state of treating pain in particular patient populations.

As always, it is wise to remember that the highest level of evidence should be used to support practice recommendations. There are three official types of information that can be used to provide information about pain management and make recommendations for practice.

1. Standards
2. Guidelines
3. Consensus statements and position papers

Often, these terms are used interchangeably and it is helpful to understand the strength of the information and the need for compliance. These types of documents are also helpful with determining what types of treatments are best for patients. When trying to decide which guideline, standard, or position paper to use in practice, the one that is most applicable to the practice with the highest level of support should be used.

1. **Standards:** Standards are often used to provide accreditation, such as those formulated by The Joint Commission or by the Commission on Accreditation of Rehabilitation Facilities (CARF). Within Joint Commission standards are requirements that specifically address how pain management should be done within a hospital setting. Standards consist of criteria established by authority or general consensus as a rule that sets the standard for quality, value, or extent (Berry et al., 2003). Do not confuse the legal term, standard of care, which determines the practice patterns of a locality, with the more general standard as defined previously (D'Arcy, 2009).
2. **Guidelines:** Guidelines are developed using a somewhat different approach than standards. A guideline is a systematic statement that is developed using an analysis of current research that indicates

which patient health care choices are appropriate for specific clinical circumstances (Berry et al., 2003). Recommendations for practice are made using an evidence-based scale that rates the research evidence from high support, usually placebo-controlled randomized studies, to lower level evidence, such as expert opinion. Examples of guidelines for pain management include the low back pain and COT guidelines from the APS.

3. **Consensus statements and position papers:** These types of statements are drafted by a society such as the ASRA to help determine appropriate approaches to practice issues for their members. They are expressions of positions or opinions of the society, academy, or organizations. The document will include expert opinion, prevailing opinion, and the existing scientific evidence (Berry et al., 2003). An example of a position paper is the ASRA position paper on the use of neuraxial analgesia and anticoagulants.

Each of the previous categories is used for different purposes. Standards set institutional requirements, guidelines examine the research and make practice recommendations, and position papers examine issues of interest to a society where a common approach to a problem is developed by the membership.

Which type of support should you use to make patient care decisions? The simple answer is whichever one fits the situation best. Position papers may provide information on how anesthesiologists use epidural catheters with orthopedic patients who are often anticoagulated with Coumadin or heparin products. For information on how to treat pain in a patient with sickle cell anemia, the APS guidelines would be best. If the questions are related to practice within an institution, a standard may direct how care is provided.

No matter what the situation, carefully examine the evidence that is being provided to support the findings. If the patient is an adult and the research support is primarily from pediatric sources, the recommendations may be suspect. Carefully review the evidence base before making a decision that might adversely affect the outcome for the patient.

The Joint Commission Requirements for Pain Management

The Joint Commission is an organization that sets standards for acute care practice. The Joint Commission focus is on patient safety, medication reconciliation, and providing a high level of care to patients and effective pain management. Every 3 years, each institution covered in the purview of The Joint Commission is surveyed, and the accreditation is renewed if the requirements are met in a satisfactory manner. Institutions who fail to meet the requirements are put on suspension and can lose their accreditation.

The information on The Joint Commission standards for pain is located in the "Provision of Care, Treatment, and Services" chapter of *The Joint Commission Manual.* Copies of the manual and frequently asked questions can be located on The Joint Commission website (www.jointcommission.org).

The four core components of the care process include:

1. Assessing patient needs;
2. Planning care, treatment, and services;
3. Providing care, treatment, and services; and
4. Coordinating care, treatment, and services. (Joint Commission Resources, 2009)

The Joint Commission standards further define the components of care that must be addressed. The care activities that need to be developed from the core components include the following:

- Providing access to levels of care and/or disciplines necessary to meet patients' needs
- Interventions based on the plan of care, including the education or instruction of patients regarding their care, treatment, and services
- Coordinating care to promote continuity when patients are referred, discharged, or transferred. (Joint Commission Resources, 2009)

What does this really mean for the hospital that needs to be compliant with The Joint Commission requirements? The immediate need is for policies and procedures to define what the hospital is going to set as policy for pain assessment. Documentation needs to be developed, and staff must be educated on how to assess and document pain. The documentation is used to record pain assessments and medication delivery. Tracking the documentation can determine if the selected treatment was effective for controlling the pain and if the best outcome was attained. The medical record system and documentation process is the substructure that provides the nurses, physicians, and other caregivers with the ways and means to manage and record the patient's pain.

Related specifically to pain management, The Joint Commission standard PC.01.02.07 states that the hospital assesses and manages the patient's pain. This is a rather open-ended requirement that makes it incumbent on every facility in Joint Commission accreditation jurisdiction to develop methods for conforming to the requirement. Most of the hospital requirements include a measure of success, such as rate of pain assessments and so forth. The specific criteria under section PC.01.02.07 include the following:

- The hospital conducts a comprehensive pain assessment that is consistent with the scope of care, treatment and services, and the patient's condition.
- The hospital uses methods to assess pain that are consistent with the patient's age, condition, and ability to understand.
- The hospital reassesses and responds to the patient's pain based on its reassessment criteria.
- The hospital either treats the patient's pain or refers the patient for treatment (Joint Commission Resources, 2009).

Every patient admitted to the hospital or seen in the emergency department of the hospital needs to have a baseline pain assessment. Because there is a mandate that the patient's age, condition, and so forth is considered, each patient must have a pain assessment that is consistent with their current ability to self report pain and any other pertinent information. This has created a need for pain assessment tools for demented and nonverbal patients, as well as translation services for the health care provider to use with non–English-speaking patients.

The documentation for this assessment can be placed on the nursing admission form or in the admitting practitioner's history and physical examination report. This assessment includes the pain intensity ratings and other aspects of a full pain assessment, such as location, duration, and mitigating factors (see Chapter 3 for the components of a complete pain assessment). Once the baseline is established, there is a need for regular pain intensity ratings and pain ratings when medication is given, to monitor the success of the chosen medication for pain. It is important that the baseline assessment be complete and pain focused if the patient is being admitted or seen with a complaint of pain.

Using an Evidence-Based Approach to Pain Management

Evidence-based practice or care consists of using research evidence to validate patient care (Summers, 2000). The nurse practitioner understands that by using the best possible evidence to guide practice, the best patient outcome should occur. In a study with 4,146 patients, those who received research-based nursing care made sizable gains in behavioral knowledge and physiologic and psychosocial outcomes when compared with those patients who received routine nursing care (Heater, Becker, & Olsen, 1988). By reviewing research-based practice recommendations, the health care provider may actually save time by eliminating those interventions that have poor support in favor of those treatments that have a higher level of research and better patient outcomes.

Practice guidelines usually contain evidence-based recommendations for treatment. Using treatments that are recommended in a guideline allows the practitioner to have confidence that they are selecting a treatment option that has been examined and proven effective at some level. This means that the guidelines should be based on a complete review of current, applicable research that is ranked to indicate the strength of the evidence and practice recommendations. Various methods sort through current research to locate the best and most usable studies, and literature review sites, such as the Cochrane Reviews (www.cochrane.org), can provide the latest and best evidence analysis of specific pain conditions. Using these research review sites can save time and reading when the salient information is summarized in the review of the topic. Several pain-related study groups in the Cochrane Review group address recommendations for interventional pain management techniques, low back pain, and complementary methods for pain management.

Always remember to assess the value of the guideline using a critical eye about the type of research used to make a recommendation for practice. If the practice recommendation is being made for adult patients who have cardiac surgery, then the research base should reflect a high number of good quality studies with adult cardiac patients.

Evaluating the strength of evidence for practice recommendation involves the use of a ranking system for studies that will determine the strength of the evidentiary support.

Strength of Evidence-Rating System

Level I: Strong

Evidence from systematic reviews, meta-analyses, and randomized clinical trials of good quality with similar results

Level II

Evidence from at least one well-constructed and well-designed randomized clinical trial

Level III

Evidence from well-designed trial without randomization

Level IV

Evidence from well-designed case control or cohort studies

Level V

Evidence from systematic reviews of descriptive or qualitative studies

Level VI

Evidence from a single descriptive or qualitative study

Level VII

Evidence derived from expert opinion or reports of expert committees (Ackley, Ladwig, Swan, & Tucker, 2008; Newhouse, Dearholt, Poe, Pugh, & White, 2007)

Practice recommendations using this type of research evaluation will rank the recommendation as strong to weak or unable to recommend.

The most comprehensive organizations with strong evidence-based support for reviewing research evidence include the following:

- The Cochrane Collaboration (http://www.cochrane.org) reviews and grades current scientific research and has several pain management study groups.
- The National Guideline Clearinghouse (http://www.guideline.gov) has a large number of clinical guidelines and is supported by the Agency for Health Care Research and Quality.
- Johanna Briggs Institute (http://www.johannabriggs.edu.au) specializes in evidence-based resources for nurses, medicine, and allied health care.

Although evidence-based practice provides superior outcomes, not all health care providers are using these recommendations, and only a small percentage incorporate research findings into patient care decisions (Melnyk, Fineout-Overholt, Stone, & Ackerman, 2000; Shorten & Wallace, 1997). When considering the use of evidence for practice decisions in general, research shows us that patients experience 28% better outcomes when research is used to drive care (Heater, Becker, & Olson, 1988).

For pain management, using evidence-based practice to treat is important because it gives the practitioner confidence in the intervention they are using for pain relief. It provides the most current information on pain medications and pain relief techniques and provides information on which items are not recommended. Evidence-based practice encourages high-quality practice, and it can improve patient outcomes. Also, the use of guidelines and evidence-based practice helps to provide the elements needed for compliance with Joint Commission requirements for pain management in acute care.

Case Study

Cindy Jones is admitted to the hospital for uncontrolled abdominal pain. She is 36 years old and has no comorbidities except for fibromyalgia. She is still in the emergency department when you are asked to see her for pain control. She tells you that the pain came on suddenly and is very intense. She does not associate the pain with an illness or exposure to a sick person. She had her period last week so doubts she is pregnant. The pain is localized to her left lower abdomen and it continues to be severe in intensity.

The emergency room nurse practitioner determines that Cindy has appendicitis and arranges for the surgeon to see her. In the meantime, Cindy is not given any pain medication, because it might mask symptoms. She waits for 4 hours in the emergency room without any pain medication and has significant pain, nausea, and vomiting. Her surgery is performed using a laparoscopic technique. Postoperatively, Cindy has difficulty getting her pain under control. She continues to complain of abdominal pain and a referred pain to her shoulder. She is only offered intermittent injections of pain medications, which make her nauseous. Because her pain is an issue, Cindy stays in the hospital for unrelieved pain and nausea. She is told that most patients with appendectomies do not have pain at her level and she should be doing better. She is converted to low-dose oral pain medications as soon as she can tolerate fluids. Her length of stay is 2 days longer than usual and Cindy is discharged from the hospital in close to the same level of pain as when she was admitted. The surgeon says he cannot understand why she continues to have unrelieved pain.

Questions to Consider

1. What would The Joint Commission say about Cindy's pain experience?
2. What guidelines or standards might apply to Cindy's care?
3. If practice recommendation from guidelines had been used to treat Cindy's condition, could her pain been controlled better and her length of stay shortened?
4. How would you provide measures of success or failure with Cindy's care for The Joint Commission?

REFERENCES

Ackley, J. B., Ladwig, G. B., Swan, B. A., & Tucker, S. J. (2008). *Evidence based nursing care guidelines: Medical-surgical interventions* (pp. 587–597). Philadelphia, PA: Mosby Elsevier.

Berry, P. H., Dahl, J., Donovan, M., Fine, P., Miaskowski, C., Stillman, M., Syrjala, K. (2003). *Improving the quality of pain management through measurement and action.* Reston, VA: National Pharmaceutical Council, Inc. and The Joint Commission.

Beyea, S., & Slattery, M. J. (2006). *Evidence-based practice in nursing: A guide to successful implementation.* Marblehead, MA: HCPro.

D'Arcy, Y. (2009). Putting pain research into practice. *Nursing 2009, 39*(8), 58.

Heater, B. S., Becker, A. M., & Olson, R. K. (1988). Nursing interventions and patient outcomes: A meta-analysis of studies. *Nursing Research, 37*(5), 303–307.

Joint Commission Resources. (2009). *CAMH 2005 Comprehensive accreditation manual for hospitals: The official handbook.* Oakbrook Terrace, IL: Author.

Marks, R. M., & Sachar, E. J. (1973). Undertreatment of medical inpatients with narcotic analgesics. *Annals of Internal Medicine, 78*(2), 173–181.

Melnyk, B. M, Fineout-Overholt, E., Stone, P., & Ackerman, M. (2000). Evidence-based practice: The past, the present, and recommendations for the millennium. *Pediatric Nursing, 26*(1), 77–80.

Newhouse, R. P., Dearholt, S. L., Poe, S. S., Pugh, L. C., & White, K. M. (2007). *Johns Hopkins nursing evidence-based practice model and guidelines.* Indianapolis, IN: Sigma Theta Tau International.

Shorten, A., & Wallace, M. (1997). Evidence-based practice. When quality counts. *Australian Nursing Journal, 4*(11), 26–27.

Summers, S. (2000). Evidence-based practice part 1: Pain definitions, pathophysiologic mechanisms, and theories. *Journal of Perianesthesia Nursing, 15*(5), 357–365.

II

Assessing Acute Pain

3

The Art and Science of Pain Assessment

OVERVIEW

Pain assessment is often considered a simple process, especially in the acute care setting. You ask the patient for a numeric rating of the pain intensity, choose a medication that will be effective for the level of pain reported, and then wait for good results. In the ideal world, everyone believes the patient's report of pain, and when you reassess the pain it has decreased and the patient is satisfied. In the real world of clinical practice, many confounding variables affect pain assessment.

Pain assessment is both an art and a science. It is one of the most challenging things that nurses, nurse practitioners, physicians, physicians' assistants, and other health care staff do in their daily practice. Assessment tools have been developed to help the health care providers obtain all the salient information needed to choose a course of treatment designed to reduce pain based on the patient's complaint. However, the health care providers still bring their own family culture, professional opinions, and experience and educational base to the process of assessment.

Pain is a difficult entity to measure and assess. It is a subjective report of a phenomenon that is a representation of the patient's experience with the pain. One person is trying to communicate to another person the intensity of a complex experience as interpreted through the patient's previous experiences with pain, the patient's expectations, and the personal response to the condition using a numeric equivalent. There are no objective tests that can provide results that indicate pain or no pain. Assessing pain is not as easy as putting on a blood pressure cuff and measuring diastolic and systolic pressure. Pain not only is the numeric intensity rating but also encompasses a wide spectrum of physiological and psychological responses that need to be considered when trying to work with the patient on a plan of care that will meet the patient's needs and produce the best outcomes.

In the acute care setting, pain assessment and adequate intervention can positively influence outcomes, such as time to discharge, participation in physical therapy, and patient satisfaction. Pain assessment and adequate management of the pain are a means to accomplish the patient and health care provider's goal of timely discharge with pain well managed. By effectively managing acute pain, patients should be able to participate in physical therapy and bring their postinjury or postsurgical activity back to their prehospital or preinjury condition. The key to adequate pain management is a comprehensive pain assessment.

Clinical Pearl

Pain assessment has been identified by health care providers as a difficult process related to the lack of objective measurement, reliance of patient's self-report of pain, lack of trust in the patient's report of pain, and use of an objective scale to convey a subjective experience. The health care provider comes to the patient interaction with bias as a result of family and personal values and beliefs about pain (D'Arcy, 2009, 2010). Using a tool such as an objective scale can help minimize some of these effects.

For the pain assessment process to be successful, the health care provider must consider the limitations of the pain assessment and look beyond the numeric rating that the patient provides. Some patients rate their pain as a 10/10—severe, but with the ability to ambulate around the nursing unit. Others rate their pain at 3/10—mild, and cannot imagine being able to get out of bed with their pain. This variance in patient reporting can lead the health care provider to misunderstand the patient's portrayal of the pain and, in some cases, lead to disbelief of the pain report.

Other patient groups are not willing to discuss their pain or the intensity of the pain. In an observational study with 270 patients with cancer, there were several concerns identified that created a barrier to assessing pain. Many of the patients in the study group had misconceptions about using opioid analgesics and feared the inability of managing side effects such as constipation and that they could become addicted to their medications (Ward et al., 1993). Additionally, some patients with cancer are afraid to report increased pain, concerned that their disease has progressed.

Some of the variation in the assessment process can be explained by lack of patient education on how to correctly rate pain intensity. Other causes are related to the patient's expectation for pain relief and the effect of the hospital experience itself. If patients believe they are too ill to move, they will tend to rate pain in a way that will prohibit activity. Some patients believe that with today's modern advances in health care, they will be pain free after surgery. This misconception can make patients feel that their expectation is not being met when they have even a mild level of pain after surgery or injury. Culture can also affect pain assessment and management. People can tend to believe that their perception and beliefs is the right viewpoint (Narayan, 2010). In order to provide the best pain assessment possible the provider must be aware of their own beliefs and then be open to differences and cultural effects in how patients perceive, describe, and react to pain.

Bias can also play a role in skewing the pain assessment process (Harrison, 1991). As health care providers, we must recognize the patients' own prejudices and opinions about the assessment process as a whole. We cannot change our own life experiences or the effect of our cultural or familial background. What we can do is to recognize that the pain is the patient's and not ours. We must respect and trust the patient's efforts to communicate pain to those that are caring for him or her. Beyond any other aspects of the pain assessment, the health care provider should believe the patient's report of pain and act on it accordingly to provide adequate pain management for the patient.

This belief of the patient's report of pain creates a trust relationship between the patient and the health care provider, which is highly beneficial to the success of the pain management plan of care.

Barriers to Pain Assessment

Some of the barriers to pain assessment were briefly mentioned in the previous section. In addition to knowledge deficits in how to rate their pain, there are other issues that interfere with getting the best possible pain assessment from patients. We are all products of our family culture and other types of thought-shaping influences that we experience as we grow up and mature.

One way to overcome bias is to use the objective measures we have in place, such as the Numeric Rating Scale (NRS) and the FACES scale, that gives us a consistent method of assessing the intensity of pain in patients in a way that can be repeated and replicated by most practitioners. Using a pain scale that is easy to use can provide a consistent measurement of the pain, which gives the health care provider a method of tracking the efficacy of pain management for the patient.

The barriers to the pain assessment process that have been identified include the following:

- *Culture and language* can be a barrier because there are subtle differences in languages that do not translate well. Some cultures do not wish to speak about pain and not discuss how to manage it. Using translated pain scales or a third party to translate can help the patient understand the pain assessment.
- The patient's *physical condition* can also be a barrier to pain assessment. If the patient is injured or pain levels are high, the patient may be unable to provide an accurate pain assessment (Munden, 2007). If pain is a barrier to pain assessment, attempt to get simple numeric rating as a start to the process and continue to reevaluate the patient using the same method.
- *Psychological condition* and *behavioral issues* can also color the pain assessment process. Anxiety and fear of pain can cause the pain assessment to be elevated. Trying to provide reassurance and medications to relieve the anxiety can make the assessment process easier.

For patients with mood disorders and psychiatric conditions, more complex assessment techniques will need to be used that include functionality, medication use, and examination of the patient's expectations.

- *Developmental ability*, *cognitive ability*, *level of consciousness*, and *the patient being nonverbal* are also significant barriers to the usual pain assessment process. In the case of the patient who cannot self-report pain, a behavioral pain scale will need to be used for the pain assessment. Later chapters in the book will provide information on the various behavioral tools that are currently being used in practice. The biggest drawback to pain assessment using a behavioral pain scale is that someone other than the patient is determining the patient's pain (Herr, Bjoro & Decker, 2006; Herr, Coyne, et al., 2006). Although the technique is not ideal, it is one way to assess pain in these individuals and, as the science becomes more refined, there may be newer techniques that are more effective. In some areas of acute care, such as critical care, stroke units, and neonatal practices, these barriers are more significant, and choosing the best pain scale to assess pain in the specific population can help decrease barriers to assessment.
- *Provider bias and knowledge deficits* about pain assessment can heavily influence the accuracy and validity of the pain assessment a health care provider performs. If the person performing the assessment perceives the patient as drug seeking or untruthful, the assessment process will result in a more negative assessment. If the prejudices and bias that all health care providers bring the practice area can be minimized, the accuracy of the pain assessment can be improved. Providing education to health care providers about how to use pain scales effectively to perform a reliable pain assessment and to choose a pain management intervention can reduce the negative effect that knowledge deficits have on the assessment process.

Although these barriers seem significant, there is currently a great deal of research being done with the various specialty populations to make sure that assessment tools meet the needs of the patient group for performing a reliable pain assessment. For the personal barriers of bias and knowledge deficits, the health care provider should become aware of the issues and develop an objective approach to the assessment process remembering that it is not their pain or their perception of pain but the patient's experience with pain that is being assessed. There are many online sites, journal articles, and educational aids that help health care providers become more proficient, consistent, and objective when assessing pain.

Elements of a Pain Assessment

The overall goal of acute pain assessment is identified as alleviating or reducing pain to a level that is acceptable to the patient (Dochterman & Bulechek, 2004). Using the elements of the pain assessment will provide the practitioner with a great deal of information about the patient's pain complaint and how the pain is affecting the patient.

Believing the patient's report of pain is critical to the success of pain assessment, many health care providers still have difficulty believing the patient's self-report of pain (Berry, Covington, Dahl, Katz, Miaskowski, 2006; D'Arcy, 2008, 2009; Donovan et al., 1987; Drayer et al., 1999; Grossman et al., 1991; Paice et al., 1991). Because pain assessment is the key to providing adequate pain management, a poor assessment or one skewed by bias or disbelief of the patient's self-report of pain can lead to untreated or undertreated pain. Studies indicate that heath care providers' fears of addicting patients, fears of respiratory depression, or an unwillingness to accept the patient's report of pain can lead to a reluctance to prescribe opioids for pain relief (Apfelbaum, 2003; Choiniere et al., 1990; D'Arcy, 2008, 2009; Donovan et al., 1987; Harrison, 1991; Marks & Scahar, 1973; Watt-Watson, 1987). Listening to the patient's report of pain, believing the report, and using the basic elements of a pain assessment can help the practitioner perform an assessment that can provide the best outcome for the patient.

Location—Have the patient point to the area on his or her body that is painful. For multiple painful areas, have the patient locate each one individually. If one area is more painful than the next, make sure the most painful area is clearly identified. If there is a radiation of pain (e.g., down a leg or arm), make sure the area is clearly defined so that the correct treatment options can be determined. A body diagram can be helpful when the patient is trying to locate the pain

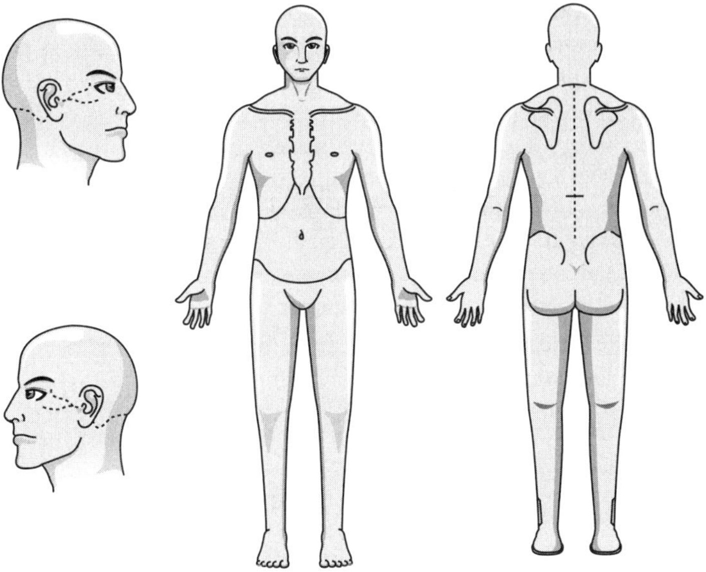

Figure 3.1 ■ Body pain diagram

(see Figure 3.1). Using colors for pain in different parts of the body can also help determine any differences in pain intensity.

Duration—Ask the patient, "When did you first feel this pain?" and "How long does the pain last?." Explore any potential sources or causes of the pain.

Intensity—Use the NRS to have the patient rate the intensity of the pain. Look for any times of the day or night when the pain intensity is more or less severe. If the patient is taking pain medication, determine how it is decreasing the pain intensity. Another option for determining pain intensity if the patient cannot use the NRS is to use the terms *mild*, *moderate*, or *severe* to see if a range for pain intensity can be determined.

Quality/Description—Have the patients describe the quality of the pain. This may be one of the most important items in the assessment process. If the patient uses words such as burning, tingling, or painful numbness, it may indicate a neuropathic source for the pain. It is important to allow the patient to describe the pain in his or her own words so it is most accurately represented.

Alleviating/Aggravating factors—All patients have some form of home treatment for pain, and they most often will attempt to treat their pain before they seek health care (Roper Starch, 2001). If the patient has tried some form of pain relief, ask if it helped (i.e., did it make the pain better or worse). Ask the patient if activity made the pain worse or if rest improved the pain.

Pain management goal—For most patients with chronic pain, the concept of pain free is not a valid goal. Work with the patient to set a goal that is reasonable and achievable. Ask the patient what pain level they think is acceptable and then tailor pain interventions to achieve the patient's expectations. Consistent pain reassessment will track progress toward the goal that has been set.

Function goal—Pain is dynamic and increases with activity (Dahl & Kehlet, 2006). Ask the patient how the pain interferes with his or her activities of daily living. Assess the patient for sleep disturbances that can affect his or her ability to function. By setting a functionality goal, progress can be tracked at each subsequent visit (D'Arcy, 2010; The Joint Commission, 2000; Pasero & McCaffery, 2004).

Although self-report is considered to be the most dependable and the gold standard for pain assessment, the process of pain assessment is a complex process (American Pain Society, 2009). When assessing the patient's pain, it is necessary to remember that the patient's self-report is covering not only the physical, sensory aspect of the pain complaint but also the emotional, psychological, and cultural response to the pain (Ackley, Ladwig, Swan, & Tucker, 2008; D'Arcy, 2010). To the patient, his or her pain is truly what he or she says it is, and it occurs when the patient says it does (McCaffery & Pasero, 1999).

From the practitioner's point of view, pain assessment is required by The Joint Commission, and many institutions have made pain assessment the "fifth vital sign." There is also discussion related to the patient's right to pain management (The Joint Commission, 2000; McDonald, 2009; Todd & Miner, 2010).

Additionally, health care practitioners are being legally challenged for the quality of their pain assessment and pain management. In a landmark case, the Estate of Henry James v. Hillhaven

Corporation was decided in favor of the plaintiff, and the court awarded $15 million to the estate for punitive and compensatory damages (Angarola & Donato, 1991). The basis of the case was undertreated pain, the documentation by the admitting nurse citing the patient as addicted to oral morphine used to control the pain of a pathological femur fracture, and the subsequent substitution of another medication for some of the morphine doses. As a direct result of the nursing assessment, the North Carolina Department of Human Resources fined the facility for patient endangerment and found the nurse liable (Pasero, 2001).

In other cases, such as William Bergman v. Wing Chin, MD and Eden Medical Center, a patient had significant pain that was undermanaged, a planned discharge from the hospital with unrelieved pain, and a documented pain score of 10/10. The patient's estate filed a civil suit, and was awarded $1.5 million in damages (reduced to $250,000) and $1 million in legal fees. The case was decided using the state of California elder abuse statutes (Rich, 2004).

There are many other legal cases in which patients did not have adequate pain management, opioid medications were misprescribed, or medical practice related to pain management was questionable. Because the assessment process is so critical to adequate and effective pain relief, performing and documenting a thorough pain assessment is a necessity for treating patients with acute pain and a process that is subject to scrutiny if the assessment is not done well or is documented poorly.

First Steps in the Assessment Process

Treating the acute care patient for pain requires a history and physical that includes the elements of pain history. The pertinent information includes the following:

- Note the patient's pain complaint, how long the pain has been present, and the elements of the pain assessment process.
- Provide a discussion of the patient's past pain experiences. This information is critical to discovering any problem areas, such as the

patients being labeled as a drug seeker or receiving inadequate pain relief during prior hospitalizations.

- Document medical history, including any conditions that can produce pain and affect pain relief, such as diabetic neuropathy or fibromyalgia. The presence of these conditions can increase the intensity of the new pain complaint. This is the patient who has high pain levels that are unexpected with even minor procedures.
- Document surgical history, including any surgeries, such as thoracotomy, where a pain condition can result such as post thoracotomy pain syndrome or phantom limb pain after amputations.
- Document psychiatric history, including any hospitalizations for mood disorders or depression.
- Review medications, including information on medications that are currently being used for pain with correct doses; medications that have been used in the past with poor effect; and those medications that have produced significant adverse effects, such as sedation, dizziness, or syncope.
- One of the biggest things that can affect pain relief in the acute care setting is patients who are actively using illicit substances or have a history of substance abuse. Unless the health care practitioner knows what substances are being used, the quantity of the substances, and how frequent the use is, pain control will be difficult if not impossible. Although the discussion can be difficult, it is imperative that the question be asked so that adequate pain medications can be provided.
- Review laboratory findings in some patients, such as in trauma patients; urine screening for drugs of abuse should be performed.
- Imaging studies will be needed and pain relief will need to be provided so that the studies can be performed effectively.
- Other relevant workups, such as electromyogram studies, should be used to determine the extent of nerve damage or other types of screening studies.

Ongoing Assessment

The pain assessment is a critical piece of the history and physical and determines what interventions are chosen for pain relief. Once the pain level has been determined through the assessment process, ongoing assessment at regular intervals can provide for the development of a comprehensive plan of care while pain is assessed with activity and ancillary symptoms such as sleep disturbances are addressed. Adjustments to the plan of care are based on the patient's response to the interventions that have been included in the plan of care (Ackley, Ladwig, Tucker, et al., 2008; Berry et al., 2006). Documentation of the pain assessment is required not only for billing purposes and insurance coverage but also to track the changes in pain intensity and the effect of the interventions.

The next two chapters will discuss pain assessment scales and tools for both standard pain assessment and pain assessment in specialty areas.

Case Study

Bob Smith is a 45-year-old truck driver on worker's compensation who has had low back pain for 5 years after a motor vehicle accident involving his truck. He is admitted to your hospital unit after undergoing back surgery. His pain assessment constantly seems to be in the severe range, 7/10–9/10, no matter what types of medication are given. The nurses are very frustrated because he requests his pain medication every time it is due but still seems to have high levels of unrelieved pain. When you ask Bob about his pain, he tells you,

> Well, you know I have been having this pain for quite a while. When I take my pain medication, I can barely make it through the day. I don't sleep well at all, and mostly I just sit in my recliner chair all night watching TV. I have tried all kinds of medications and physical therapies, but the doctor said the surgery was the only thing that would help, so I agreed to have it. Now since the surgery the pain is so much worse and I can scarcely get up out of bed. Will it always be this way? I would love to have good pain relief and get off those pain medications.

His medication regimen is extended-release oxycodone, 240 mg twice per day and 20 mg of oxycodone for breakthrough pain that he has been taking for the past 6 months. He also drinks a 12 pack of beer every week and occasionally smokes marijuana.

Questions to Consider

1. What type of pain assessment tool would be best for Bob?
2. What elements of the pain assessment are coming out as the most important aspect of Bob's pain complaint?
3. Does the chronic pain that Bob has had over the past 5 years affect his current pain assessment?
4. Do you think Bob should be considered as drug seeking or addicted to his pain medications?
5. One of the nurses keeps telling you that she cannot believe his pain is still so severe and that he must be making it up. What do you tell the nurse about a patient like Bob and his pain assessment?

REFERENCES

Ackley, B., Ladwig, G., Swan, B. A., & Tucker, S. J. (2008). *Evidence-based nursing care guidelines.* St. Louis, MO: Mosby Elsevier.

American Pain Society. (2009). *Principles of analgesic use in the treatment of acute and cancer pain* (5th ed). Glenview, IL: Author.

Angarola, R. T., & Donato, B. J. (1991). Inappropriate pain management results in high jury award. *Journal of Pain and Symptom Management, 6*(7), 407.

Apfelbaum, J., Chen, C., Mehta, S., & Tong, G. (2003). Postoperative pain experience: Results from a national survey suggest postoperative pain continues to be undermanaged. *Anesthesia & Analgesia, 97*(2), 534–540.

Berry, P. H., Covington, E., Dahl, J., Katz, J., & Miaskowski, C. (2006). *Pain: Current understanding of assessment, management, and treatments.* Reston, VA: National Pharmaceutical Council, Inc.

Choinière, M., Melzack, R., Girard, N., Rondeau, J., & Pacquin, M. J. (1989). Comparisons between patients' and nurses' assessment of pain and medication efficacy in severe burn injuries. *Pain, 40*(2), 143–152.

Dahl, J. B., & Kehlet, H. (2006). Postoperative pain and its management. In S. B. McMahon & M. Kolzenburg (Eds.), *Wall & Melzack's textbook of pain* (5th ed.). Philadelphia, PA: Churchill Livingstone.

D'Arcy, Y. (2007). *Pain management: Evidence-based tools and techniques for nursing professionals.* Marblehead, MA: HCPro.

D'Arcy, Y. (2008). Nursing 2008 pain management survey report. *Nursing, 38*(6), 42–49.

D'Arcy, Y. (2009). Be in the know about pain management. Results of the pain management survey. *The Nurse Practitioner, 34*(4), 43–47.

D'Arcy, Y. (2010). *Core curriculum for pain management nursing* (2nd ed.). Dubuque, IA: Kendall-Hunt Professional.

Dochterman, J. M., & Bulechek, G. M. (Eds.). (2004). *Nursing interventions classification (NIC)* (4th ed.). St. Louis, MO: Mosby.

Donovan, M., Dillon, P., & McGuire, L. (1987). Incidence and characteristics of pain in a sample of medical-surgical inpatients. *Pain, 30*(1), 69–78.

Drayer, R. A., Henderson, J., & Reidenberg, M. (1999). Barriers to better pain control in hospitalized patients. *Journal of Pain and Symptom Management, 17*(6), 434–440.

Grossman, S. A., Scheidler, V., Swedeen, K., Mucenski, J., & Piantadosi, S. (1991). Correlation of patient and caregiver ratings of cancer pain. *Journal of Pain and Symptom Management, 6*(2), 53–57.

Harrison, A. (1991). Assessing patients' pain: Identifying reasons for error. *Journal of Advanced Nursing, 16*(9), 1018-1025.

Herr, K., Bjoro, K., & Decker, S. (2006). Tools for assessment of pain in nonverbal older adults with dementia: A state-of-the-science review. *Journal of Pain and Symptom Management, 31*(2), 170–192.

Herr, K., Coyne, P. J., Key, T., Manworren, R., McCaffery, M., Merkel, S., . . . Wild, L. (2006). Pain assessment in the nonverbal patient: Position statement with clinical practice recommendations. *Pain Management Nursing, 7*(2), 44–52.

The Joint Commission. (2000). *Pain assessment and management: An organizational approach*. Oakbrook Terrace, IL: Author.

Marks, R., Sachar, E. (1973). Undertreatment of medical inpatients with narcotic analgesics. *Annals of Internal Medicine, 78,* 173–181.

McCaffery, M., & Pasero, C. (1999). *Pain: Clinical manual* (2nd ed.). St. Louis, MO: Mosby.

Munden, J. (Ed.). (2007). *Best practices: Evidence-based nursing procedures.* Philadelphia, PA: Lippincott Williams & Wilkins.

Narayan, M. C. (2010). Culture's effects on pain assessment and management. *American Journal of Nursing, 110*(4), 38–47.

Paice, J., Mahon, S. M., & Faut-Callahan, M. (1991). Factors associated with adequate pain control in hospitalized postsurgical patients diagnosed with cancer. *Cancer Nursing, 14*(6), 298–305.

Pasero, C., & McCaffery, M. (2001). The Undertreatment of Pain. *American Journal of Nursing, 101*(11), 62–65.

Pasero, C., & McCaffery, M. (2004). Comfort-function goals: A way to establish accountability for pain relief. *American Journal of Nursing, 104*(9), 77–78.

Rich, B. A. (2004). Thinking the unthinkable: The clinician as perpetrator of elder abuse in patients in pain. *Journal of Pain and Palliative Care Pharmacotherapy, 18*(3), 63–74.

Roper Starch Worldwide, Inc. (1999). *Chronic pain in America: Roadblocks to relief.* Available at www.painfoundation.org/page.asp?file

Todd, K., & Miner, R. (2010). In J. D. Loeser et al. (Eds.), *Bonica's management of pain.* Philadelphia, PA: Lippincott Williams & Wilkins.

Ward, S. E., Goldberg, N., Miller-McCauley, V., Mueller, C., Nolan, A., Pawlik-Plank, D., . . . Weissman, D. E. (1993). Patient-related barriers to the management of cancer pain. *Pain, 52*(3), 319–324.

Watt-Watson, J. (1987). Nurses' knowledge of pain issues: A survey. *Journal of Pain and Symptom Management, 2*(4), 207–211.

4

Assessment Tools for Acute Pain

OVERVIEW OF ASSESSMENT TOOLS

There are various tools for assessing acute pain. Some tools are widely used for general pain assessment and others are designed for specific populations, such as children, nonverbal adults, or intubated critically ill patients. This chapter will provide information on the tools used to assess pain in the general population and provide hints for performing a pain assessment on a patient with acute pain.

The use of a numeric rating for pain intensity is just the beginning of the assessment process. The numeric pain rating does provide a means of measuring the efficacy of a medication or intervention that has been chosen to treat the pain. If the number decreases after medication is administered or a pain relief option such as massage or relaxation is performed, then the number indicates that the intervention decreased the pain. Because the efficacy of the intervention is helpful in determining if the chosen modality is working, a single-item pain assessment tool can be used.

There are also tools that have been developed for assessing chronic pain. These tools are multidimensional and are designed to measure pain intensity, medication efficacy, and functionality. These are more commonly used in the outpatient setting. Information on tools to assess chronic pain can be found in the *Compact Clinical Guide to Chronic Pain Management: An Evidence-Based Approach for Nurses* (Springer Publishing Company, 2011). The tools discussed in this book will relate specifically to acute pain assessment.

One-Dimensional Pain Assessment Tools

Some of the one-dimensional pain assessment tools, such as the visual analog scale (VAS), were developed for research and others, such as the numeric rating scale (NRS), have developed through clinical use. One-dimensional pain assessment tools for the general patient population are limited to assessing the single element of pain intensity. These tools include VAS, verbal descriptor scale (VDS), NRS, and the combined thermometer scale.

In the acute care setting, the one-dimensional scales are most helpful for determining the effectiveness of a pain medication or a pain intervention in reducing the intensity of the pain. Although these tools seem very simple and the information obtained is limited, there definitely is a place for them in pain assessment. In a review of 164 journal articles on pain assessment, single-item ratings of pain intensity were reported as valid and reliable indicators of pain intensity (Jensen, 2003). As an indication of efficacy, Farrar, Young, LaMoreaux, Werth, and Poole (2001) determined that a 2-point or 30% reduction in pain intensity on the NRS is a clinically significant change.

When assessing a patient for acute pain who also has a chronic pain condition, it is good practice to determine what the patient's baseline pain intensity from the chronic pain is on a daily basis. To get a good indication of the pain intensity that the patient has daily, ask the patient what the best pain intensity is during the day, what the worst pain intensity is, and what the average pain intensity is for any given day or a particular time of day. For a patient with chronic pain, a daily pain rating of 4–5 may be what can best be achieved with the patient's usual medications. When the patient has acute pain on top of chronic pain, getting the pain rating below the daily best pain score level will be difficult, if not impossible. For this type of patient, continuing or restarting the usual pain medication and setting a pain goal that is close to the best daily pain rating will set a target that the health care practitioner can work toward. Discharge from the hospital should not be postponed if this type of patient has an increased pain rating, as long as adequate pain relief is being provided, and such patients indicate they had elevated pain scores before hospitalization.

The Joint Commission (2000) mandates that all patients admitted to a hospital have their pain assessed and reassessed regularly. Most hospitals use a 0–10 Likert-type NRS that can quickly assess pain intensity. It is always a good idea to assess the patient's pain while the patient is immobile in bed and also with activity. Pain is dynamic and will increase with activity (Dahl & Kehlet, 2006). For some patients who are admitted through the Emergency Room the full comprehensive admission pain assessment will be performed in the ER. For other patients the admission database will contain the full pain assessment while in outpatient practice the first visit history and physical will be where the documentation of the full pain assessment will be located.

For nonverbal patients or patients in special categories, a behavioral scale using pain indicators is more appropriate; these scales will be discussed in Chapter 5. Each hospital sets standards for daily pain assessments and additionally has a policy for pain assessment and reassessment when medications are administered. A typical policy of reassessing pain after medication delivery would be to reassess pain after oral medication in an hour and for intravenous (IV) medications at 30 minutes. Medication adjustments may be needed if pain intensity ratings remain high.

There are various one-dimensional pain assessment tools that can be used for assessing pain in acute care. Some, such as VAS, are more commonly used in research, but others, such as the NRS, are commonly used for clinical pain assessments since they are easy for patients to understand and for health care providers to use and score.

Visual Analog Scale (VAS)

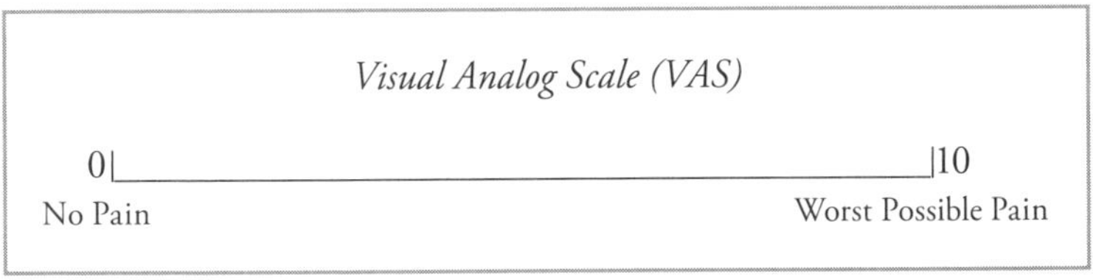

The VAS is a 100-mm line with "no pain" at one end and "worst pain possible" at the other end. The tool was designed to be used for research in which a mark on the line could easily be measured to ascertain the intensity of the pain. To use the VAS, the health care provider asks the patients to mark on the 100-mm line where they feel their pain intensity would be represented. If a patient marks the line at the 50-mm position, the pain would be 5/10 when compared to the NRS, or a moderate level pain.

The VAS is one of the most basic scales and has some limitations for clinical use.

Limitations to this scale include the following:

- Some older adult patients have difficulty marking on the line and place the mark above or below the 100-mm line (Herr & Garand, 2001; Herr & Mobily, 1993).
- Reassessment and comparison options are limited (D'Arcy, 2010).

Verbal Descriptor Scale (VDS)

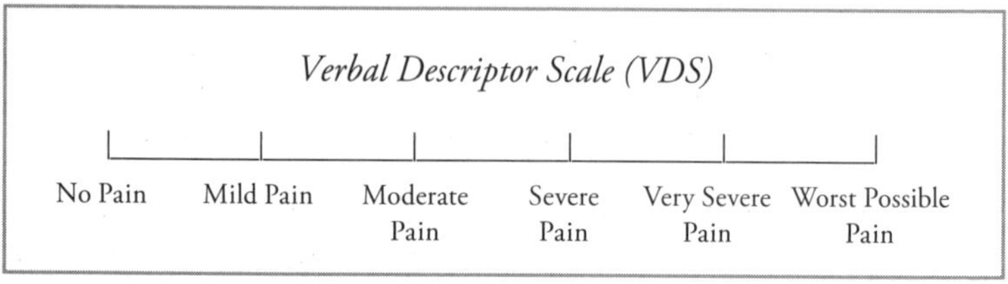

The VDS allows patients to use word descriptors to rate their pain. The scale is anchored on one end with "no pain" and on the other end with "worst pain possible." The words mild, moderate, and severe are used to measure pain intensity. To use the scale, the nurse asks the patients to select the word that best describes the pain they are experiencing. Clinically, some patients prefer to use a word to describe their pain rather than a number. Although normally used for cognitively intact patients, Feldt, Ryden, and Miles (1998) found a 73% completion rate with the VDS in cognitively impaired patients.

Limitations to this pain scale include the following:

- The patient must be able to understand the meaning of the words.
- Reassessment and comparisons are difficult (D'Arcy, 2010).

Numeric Rating Scale (NRS)

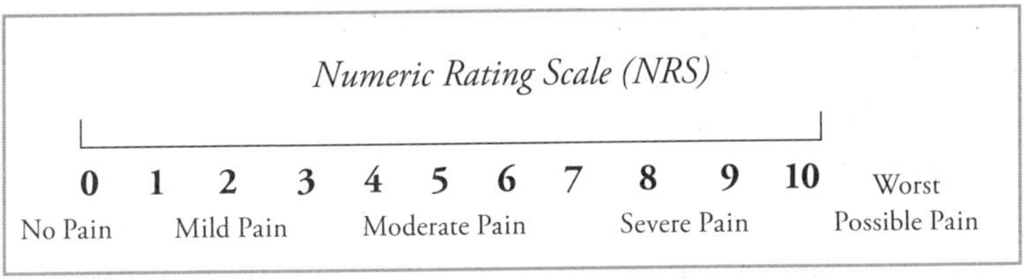

The NRS is the most commonly used one-dimensional pain scale. It is an 11-point Likert-type scale where 0 means "no pain" and 10 means "worst possible pain." To use the scale, the health care provider asks the patient to rate his or her pain intensity from 0–10. The higher the number, the more intense the pain.

Mild pain is considered to be pain ratings in the 1–3 range.
Moderate pain is considered to be pain ratings in the 4–6 range.
Severe pain is considered to be pain ratings in the 7–10 range.

Although there is discussion about whether a single number rating of pain is accurate, the data indicate that single-item ratings can be useful, and the numeric rating can also be used to determine if the medication or intervention being used for pain control is effectively relieving the pain. There is no good or bad, wrong or right number for the patient to report. It is important to believe the report of pain that the patient provides. Patient self-report is still considered the gold standard for pain assessment (American Pain Society [APS], 2008). Limitation:

- Only measures one aspect of pain, intensity

Strengths:

- Allows for reassessment and comparison of pain scores
- Simple format that is easy for most patients to use (D'Arcy, 2010)

Combined Thermometer Scale

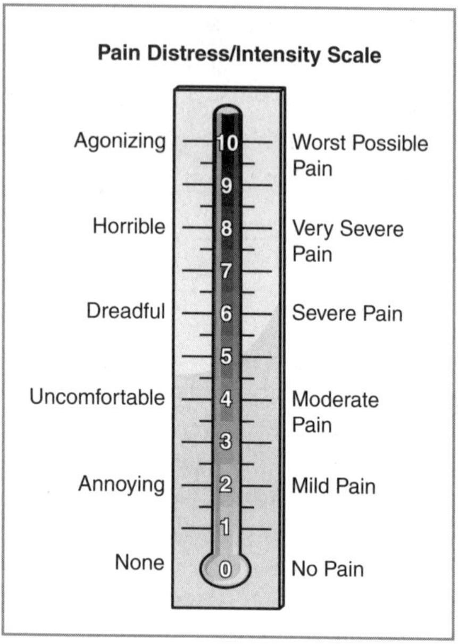

Some patients do well when they can see a graphic pain scale. The Combined Thermometer Scale[1] combines one-dimensional scales: the VDS and the NRS. Some patients like the vertical orientation where the numbers increase from the bottom upward. If colors are used, starting with 0 being blue and increasing to 10 as red also conveys increasing pain in a visual sense to the patient. This scale also has some descriptors that can indicate the effect of the pain on the patient by asking how much distress the pain is causing.

Strengths:

- Able to replicate pain ratings for reassessment
- Simple and easy-to-use format (D'Arcy, 2010)

[1]The Combined Thermometer Scale appears in color on the inside front cover.

ASSESSING PAIN USING A PAIN ASSESSMENT TOOL AS AN INTERVIEW

Brief Pain Impact Questionnaire (BPIQ)

The Brief Pain Impact Questionnaire (BPIQ) is a pain assessment tool designed as an interview. For the initial pain assessment, the health care provider will find that this tool provides a comprehensive assessment of pain, along with questions about pain history and medication use. For health care providers, using this type of an interview format can help develop a pain focused history and physical. Although it is a good tool to use for outpatients, it can also be adapted for areas of the acute care setting where a more comprehensive pain assessment is needed or for patients who are having difficulty getting adequate pain control. This tool can provide additional information for a history and physical and can also open a discussion about pain medication use, functionality, and substance abuse.

Brief Pain Impact Questionnaire (BPIQ)

- How strong is your pain right now? Is it worse or average compared to the pain you've experienced during the past week?
- How many days during the past week have you been unable to do what you would like to do because of your pain?
- During the past week, how often has pain interfered with your ability to take care of yourself? For example, has it interfered with bathing, eating, dressing, and going to the toilet?
- Over the past week, how often has pain interfered with your ability to take care of your home-related chores such as grocery shopping, preparing meals, paying bills, and driving?
- How often do you participate in pleasurable activities such as hobbies, socializing with friends, and travel? Over the past week, how often has pain interfered with these activities?
- How often do you do some type of exercise? Over the past week, how often has pain interfered with your ability to exercise?

(Continued)

(Continued)

- Does pain interfere with your ability to think clearly?
- Does pain interfere with your appetite? Have you lost weight?
- Does pain interfere with your sleep? How often over the last week has pain kept you awake at night?
- Has pain interfered with your energy, mood, personality, or relationships with other people?
- Over the past week, have you taken pain medications?
- Has your use of alcohol or other drugs ever caused a problem for you or those close to you?
- How would you rate your health at the present time? (Weiner, Herr, & Rudy, 2002)

Source: Used with permission of the author.

Case Study

Peter Smith, 32 years of age, is an electrician who is being seen in the emergency department. He has fallen from a ladder while at work and is complaining of severe level, 8/10 side and back pain. He remembers the fall and does not think he lost consciousness. His fall was from at least 20 feet, and the owner of the property called 911 to transport Peter to the hospital. On admission to the emergency room, Peter has stable vital signs and no apparent injuries. He complains of back pain, so he is sent for a computed tomography (CT) scan to determine if there is any fracture. The CT scan reports show that there is a compression fracture in Peter's lumbar spine and two fractured ribs. Peter continues to complain of pain and was given an IV opioid to help relieve the pain.

Questions to Consider

1. Is the numeric pain rating Peter provided sufficient to assess his pain?
2. Peter is rating his pain in the severe level, 8/10. Is the IV medication a good choice or should Peter be given something oral or an NSAID? (See Pain Protocol in the Medication Section, Section III.)
3. Peter is being given IV medications for pain. How long should the nurse wait to reassess Peter's pain?
4. Would any of the other one-dimensional pain scales be more appropriate to assess Peter's pain or is the NRS the best choice?

REFERENCES

American Pain Society. (2003). *Principles of analgesic use in the treatment of acute and cancer pain* (5th ed.). Glenview, IL: Author.

Dahl, J. B., & Kehlet, H. (2006). Postoperative pain and its management. In S. B. McMahon & M. Kolzenburg (Eds.), *Wall & Melzack's textbook of pain* (5th ed.). Philadelphia, PA: Churchill Livingstone.

D'Arcy, Y. (2010). *Core curriculum for pain management nursing* (2nd ed.). Dubuque, IA: Kendall Hunt Professional.

Farrar, J. T., Young, J. P., Jr., LaMoreaux, L., Werth, J. L., & Poole, R. M. (2001). Clinical importance of changes in chronic pain intensity measured on an 11-point numerical pain rating scale. *Pain, 94*, 149–158.

Feldt, K. S., Ryden, M. B., & Miles, S. (1998). Treatment of pain in cognitively impaired compared with cognitively intact older patients with hip fracture. *Journal of the American Geriatrics Society, 46*, 1079–1085.

Herr, K. A., & Mobily, P. R. (1993). Comparison of selected pain assessment tools for use with the elderly. *Applied Nursing Research, 6*(1), 39–46.

Herr, K. A., & Garand, L. (2001). Assessment and measurement of pain in older adults. *Clinics in Geriatric Medicine, 17*(3), 457–478.

Jensen, M. P. (2003). The validity and reliability of pain measures in adults with cancer. *The Journal of Pain, 4*(1), 2–21.

The Joint Commission Resources. (2000). *Pain assessment and management: An organizational approach.* Oakbrook Terrace, IL: Author.

Weiner, D. K., Herr, K., & Rudy, T. E. (2002). *Persistent pain in older adults: An interdisciplinary guide for treatment.* New York, NY: Springer.

5

Assessing Pain in Specialty Populations

ACUTE PAIN ASSESSMENT

For most patients with acute pain, a simple Numeric Rating Scale (NRS) assessment using the 0 to 10 pain intensity will be sufficient. There are some patient populations where a more detailed or specialized pain assessment is needed. For these patient groups, there are pain assessment scales and tools that can make the assessment process easier and more consistent.

MULTIDIMENSIONAL PAIN SCALES FOR PATIENTS WITH UNDERLYING CHRONIC PAIN CONDITIONS

Some patients being seen, either in the hospital or in the outpatient clinic with an acute pain complaint, may have an underlying chronic pain condition that makes it more difficult to perform a pain assessment. Using a tool for assessing the chronic pain can help resolve some of the questions that the health care provider may have about why pain ratings seem to be consistently high with this patient group. Separating the two types of pain may be useful for making decisions about treatment options.

Multidimensional scales are used to assess patients with chronic pain with various pain conditions. The two scales that are most often used in the clinical setting for adults are the McGill Pain Questionnaire (MPQ) and the Brief Pain Inventory (BPI). The difference between the one-dimensional and the multidimensional scales is the combination of indexes in the multidimensional scale that provide the following:

- Pain intensity assessment
- Mood assessment
- A body diagram to locate pain
- Verbal descriptors
- Medication efficacy questions

When the patient rates his or her pain using a multidimensional pain scale, there is the opportunity for the patient to more completely convey the pain experience to the health care provider. The mood scales on some multidimensional scales can help define the impact of the continued pain on the patient's personal life and relationships.

McGill Pain Questionnaire (MPQ)

The MPQ was designed to be used for pain that requires a multidimensional approach to measure pain in patients with complex pain conditions, such as chronic pain. Some of the areas in which the pain scale has been used include the following:

- Experimentally induced pain
- Postprocedural pain
- A number of medical–surgical conditions

The tool contains a visual analog scale (VAS), a present pain intensity (PPI) scale, and a set of verbal descriptors used to capture the sensory aspect of the pain experience. The tool has been widely used in various settings and found to be reliable and valid and has been translated into several foreign languages (Chok, 1998; Graham, Bond, Gerkovich, & Cook, 1980; McDonald & Weiskopf, 2001; McIntyre et al., 1995; Melzack, 1975, 1987; Mystakidou et al., 2002; Wilkie, 1990).

McGill Pain Questionnaire (MPQ)–Short Form

PATIENT'S NAME: _____ DATE: _____

	NONE	MILD	MODERATE	SEVERE
THROBBING	0) _____	1) _____	2) _____	3) _____
SHOOTING	0) _____	1) _____	2) _____	3) _____
STABBING	0) _____	1) _____	2) _____	3) _____
SHARP	0) _____	1) _____	2) _____	3) _____
CRAMPING	0) _____	1) _____	2) _____	3) _____
GNAWING	0) _____	1) _____	2) _____	3) _____
HOT/BURNING	0) _____	1) _____	2) _____	3) _____
ACHING	0) _____	1) _____	2) _____	3) _____
HEAVY	0) _____	1) _____	2) _____	3) _____
TENDER	0) _____	1) _____	2) _____	3) _____
SPLITTING	0) _____	1) _____	2) _____	3) _____
TIRING/EXHAUSTING	0) _____	1) _____	2) _____	3) _____
SICKENING	0) _____	1) _____	2) _____	3) _____
FEARFUL	0) _____	1) _____	2) _____	3) _____
PUNISHING/CRUEL	0) _____	1) _____	2) _____	3) _____

VAS NO PAIN |—————————————————————————| WORST POSSIBLE PAIN

PPI

0 NO PAIN _____
1 MILD _____
2 DISCOMFORTING _____
3 DISTRESSING _____
4 HORRIBLE _____
5 EXCRUCIATING _____

© R. Melzack 1984

The short-form McGill Pain Questionnaire (SF-MPQ). Descriptors 1–11 represent the sensory dimension of pain experience and 12–15 represent the affective dimension. Each descriptor is ranked on an intensity scale of 0 = none, 1 = mild, 2 = moderate, 3 = severe. The Present Pain Intensity (PPI) of the standard long-form McGill Pain Questionnaire (LF-MPQ) and the visual analogue scale (VAS) are also included to provide overall intensity scores. Used by permission of the author.

Source: Reprinted with permission from R. Melzack. © R. Melzack, 1984.

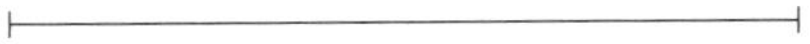

Strength:

- High level of reliability and validity

Limitations:

- Difficulty scoring and weighting the verbal descriptor section
- Difficulty translating the verbal descriptor section into words that indicate syndromes (Gracely & Dubner, 1987; Graham et al., 1980)

More recent revision of the MPQ, the SF-MPQ-2, not only includes the standard McGill questions but also includes a subscale that can determine whether pain is neuropathic or nociceptive (Dworkin et al., 2009). This recent revision allows the health care provider who is assessing a chronic pain condition to use the pain assessment to help determine the appropriate medication choices by identifying the source of the pain.

Brief Pain Inventory (BPI)

Originally, the BPI was first used with patients diagnosed with cancer to assess long-term oncology pain. With further use, it has been found to be reliable and valid for assessing pain in patients with chronic pain (Daut, Cleeland, & Flanery, 1983; Raiche et al., 2006; Tittle et al., 2003; Tan et al., 2004; Williams, Smith, & Fehnel, 2006) and has been translated into various languages (Ger, Ho, Sun, Wang, & Cleeland, 1999; Klepstad et al., 2002; Mystakidou et al., 2002; Radbruch et al., 1999). It has a simple and easy-to-use format that can be used as an interview or as a self-report that is completed by the patient. The BPI includes the following:

- A pain intensity scale
- A body diagram to locate the pain
- A functional assessment
- Questions about the efficacy of pain medications

Strength:

- High level of reliability and validity

Brief Pain Inventory

STUDY ID #: __________ DO NOT WRITE ABOVE THIS LINE HOSPITAL #: __________

Date: ____/____/____ Time: _______

Name: ____________________ ____________________ ____________________
Last First Middle Initial

1. Throughout our lives, most of us have had pain from time to time (such as minor headaches, sprains, and toothaches). Have you had pain other than these every-day kinds of pain today?

   1. Yes 2. No

2. On the diagram, shade in the areas where you feel pain. Put an X on the area that hurts the most.

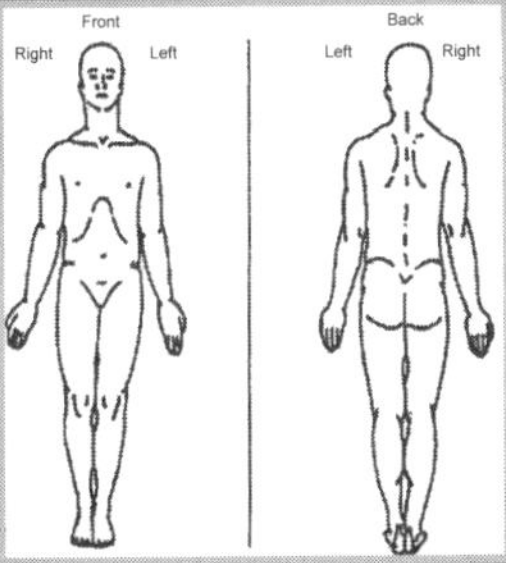

3. Please rate your pain by circling the one number that best describes your pain at its **worst** in the last 24 hours.

0 No Pain	1	2	3	4	5	6	7	8	9	10 Pain as bad as you can imagine

4. Please rate your pain by circling the one number that best describes your pain at its **least** in the last 24 hours.

0 No Pain	1	2	3	4	5	6	7	8	9	10 Pain as bad as you can imagine

5. Please rate your pain by circling the one number that best describes your pain on the **average.**

0 No Pain	1	2	3	4	5	6	7	8	9	10 Pain as bad as you can imagine

6. Please rate your pain by circling the one number that tells how much pain you have **right now.**

0 No Pain	1	2	3	4	5	6	7	8	9	10 Pain as bad as you can imagine

Page 1 of 2

(Continued)

STUDY ID #:__________ DO NOT WRITE ABOVE THIS LINE HOSPITAL #: __________

Date: ____/____/____ Time: ________

Name: __________________ __________________ ________________
Last First Middle Initial

7. What treatments or medications are you receiving for your pain?

8. In the last 24 hours, how much relief have pain treatments or medications provided? Please circle the one percentage that most shows how much relief you have received.

0% No Relief	10%	20%	30%	40%	50%	60%	70%	80%	90%	100% Complete Relief

9. Circle the one number that describes how, during the past 24 hours, pain has interfered with your:

A. General Activity

0 Does not Interfere	1	2	3	4	5	6	7	8	9	10 Completely Interferes

B. Mood

0 Does not Interfere	1	2	3	4	5	6	7	8	9	10 Completely Interferes

C. Walking Ability

0 Does not Interfere	1	2	3	4	5	6	7	8	9	10 Completely Interferes

D. Normal Work (includes both work outside the home and housework)

0 Does not Interfere	1	2	3	4	5	6	7	8	9	10 Completely Interferes

E. Relations with other people

0 Does not Interfere	1	2	3	4	5	6	7	8	9	10 Completely Interferes

F. Sleep

0 Does not Interfere	1	2	3	4	5	6	7	8	9	10 Completely Interferes

G. Enjoyment of life

0 Does not Interfere	1	2	3	4	5	6	7	8	9	10 Completely Interferes

Page 2 of 2

Source: Used with permission of the author

Limitations for the BPI include the following:

- The patients must be able to answer questions related to their individual chronic pain conditions.

Behavioral Pain Scales

As of 2001, The Joint Commission applied pain standards to inpatient care that have set a standard for outpatient practice as well. One of the biggest focus areas in The Joint Commission standards was pain assessment for all patients that included assessing pain in individuals who could not self-report their pain. To facilitate the process, a group of pain assessment tools have been developed to use for assessing pain in the nonverbal patient.

The use of behavioral scales for pain assessment is one of the newest areas of focus for pain assessment and as such, the tools that are used are not as refined or completely developed as those that have been used for many years. The current tools are not ideal, but they are the best that we have to use at this time. Some of the tools are designed to be used for specific populations, such as demented patients or critically ill intubated patients.

To use a behavioral scale, it is important to identify those behaviors that indicate pain. The original research in this area was to develop a list of behaviors that were indicative of pain, the Checklist of Nonverbal Pain Indicators (CNPI). From the studies comparing pain in cognitively intact patients and similar pain experiences in patients who were cognitively impaired, a list of six behaviors was developed to indicate the presence of pain (Feldt, 2000; Feldt, Ryden, & Miles, 1998). The six behaviors were identified as follows:

1. Vocalizations
2. Facial grimacing
3. Bracing
4. Rubbing
5. Restlessness
6. Vocal complaints (Feldt, 2000)

Additional behaviors that were determined to be indicative of pain were listed in the American Geriatrics Society's (AGS; 2002) guideline for treating persistent pain in older persons. These behaviors include the following:

- Verbalizations: moaning, calling out, asking for help, groaning
- Facial expressions: grimacing, frowning, wrinkled forehead, distorted expressions
- Body movements: rigid tense body posture, guarding, rocking, fidgeting, pacing, massaging the painful area
- Changes in interpersonal interactions: aggression, combative behavior, resisting care, disruptive, withdrawn
- Changes in activity patterns or routines: refusing food, appetite changes, increase in rest or sleep, increased wandering
- Mental status changes: crying, tears, increased confusion, irritability, or distress (AGS, 2002)

When attempting to assess pain in a nonverbal patient, the important elements include the following:

- Attempt a self-report.
- Search for the potential causes of pain.
- Observe patient behaviors.
- Use surrogate reporting by family or caregivers indicating pain and/or behavior and activity changes.
- Attempt an analgesic trial. (Herr et al., 2006)

To use behaviors to identify pain, tools have been developed using the behaviors and formatting the assessment in several different styles to use in different patient populations.

Behavioral Pain Scale for Adults

When the patients cannot self-report their pain, a behavioral pain assessment tool is needed. The Behavioral Pain Scale (BPS) was developed for such use, and it can be adapted for scoring on a 0 to 10 pain scale rating. This tool uses five categories to assess for pain with three possible ratings: 0, normal; 1, present; 2, highly visible.

Behavioral Pain Scale (Nonverbal) for Patients Unable to Provide a Self Report of Pain

	0	1	2	
Face	Face muscles relaxed.	Facial muscle tension, frown, grimace.	Frequent to constant frown, clenched jaw.	**Face Score:**
Restlessness	Quiet, relaxed appearance, normal movement.	Occasional restless movement, shifting position.	Frequent restless movement may include extremities or head.	**Restlessness Score:**
Muscle Tone*	Normal muscle tone, relaxed.	Increased tone, flexion of fingers and toes.	Rigid tone.	**Muscle Tone Score:**
Vocalization**	No abnormal sounds.	Occasional moans, cries, whimpers, or grunts.	Frequent or continuous moans, cries, whimpers, or grunts.	**Vocalization Score:**
Consolability	Content, relaxed.	Reassured by touch or talk. Distractible.	Difficult to comfort by touch or talk.	**Consolability Score:**

Behavioral Pain Assessment Scale Total (0–10)

Developed by Margaret Campbell, Detroit Receiving Hospital
*Assess muscle tone in patients with spinal cord lesion or injury at a level above the lesion or injury. Assess patients with hemiplegia on the unaffected side.
** This item cannot be measured in patients with artificial airways.

(Continued)

(Continued)

How to Use the Pain Assessment Behavioral Scale:

1. Observe behaviors and mark appropriate number for each category.
2. Total the numbers in the Pain Assessment Behavioral Score column.
3. Zero = no evidence of pain; Mild pain = 1–3; Moderate pain = 4–5; Severe uncontrolled pain is ≥ 6.

Considerations:

1. Use the standard pain scale whenever possible to obtain the patient's self-report of pain. Self-report is the best indicator of the presence and intensity of pain.
2. Use this scale for patients who are unable to provide a self-report of pain.
3. In addition, a "proxy pain evaluation" from family, friends, or clinicians close to the patient may be helpful to evaluate pain based on previous knowledge of patient response.
4. When in doubt, provide an analgesic. "If there is reason to suspect pain, an analgesic trial can be diagnostic as well as therapeutic."

Source: Used with permission of the author.

1. Facial expression
2. Restlessness
3. Vocalization
4. Muscle tension
5. Consolability

The tool is simple and easy to use in the acute care setting and has been studied for reliability and validity. It also provides a means of consistently assessing pain in patients who cannot self-report pain.

Pain Assessment in Advanced Dementia

Demented individuals are some of the most difficult patient to assess for pain. Many are nonverbal, and determining pain by behaviors can be challenging. The Pain Assessment Tool in Advanced Dementia (PAINAD) is a pain assessment tool created to assess pain in patients with advanced dementia and Alzheimer's disease (Lane et al., 2003; Warden, Hurley, & Volicer, 2003).

PAINAD

Score	0	1	2
Breathing	Normal	Occasional labored breathing, short period of hyperventilation	Noisy labored breathing, long period of hyperventilation, Cheyne-Stokes respirations
Negative Vocalization	None	Occasional moan/groan, low-level speech/negative or disapproving quality	Repeated troubled calling out, loud moaning or groaning, crying
Facial Expression	Smiling/inexpressive	Sad, frightened, frown	Facial grimacing
Body Language	Relaxed	Tense, distressed pacing, fidgeting	Rigid, fists clenched, knees pulled up, pulling or pushing away, striking out
Consolability	No need to console	Distracted or reassured by voice or touch	Unable to console, distract, or reassure

Total _____

Source: Developed at the New England Geriatric Research Education and Clinical Center, EN Rogers Memorial Veterans Hospital, Bedford, MA. From "Development and psychometric evaluation of the Pain Assessment in Advanced Dementia (PAINAD) Scale," by V. Warden, A. C. Hurley, and L. Volicer, 2003, *Journal of the American Medical Directors Association, 4*, 9–15.

The PAINAD uses five behaviors common to patients with dementia who have pain.

1. Breathing
2. Negative vocalizations
3. Facial expression
4. Body language
5. Consolability

To use the tool, the five behaviors are rated as follows:

- **0**—Normal, no symptoms or pain behaviors
- **1**—Occasional, slightly affected (e.g., occasional pacing, occasional moans)
- **2**—Positive behaviors (e.g., hyperventilation, body rigidity, repeated moaning or striking out)

After determining the extent of the behaviors, they are rated and a score is derived, providing a numeric rating for the pain. Using this tool can provide a more consistent approach to assessing pain in these patients. The tool has been found to be simple and easy to use in the clinical setting (Hutchinson et al., 2006). It has also resulted in increased detection of pain (Hutchinson et al.). Limitations include the following:

- Caregiver assesses for pain.
- Less comprehensive than needed for assessing pain (Herr, Bjoro, & Decker, 2006)

There are other tools that can be used in this patient population to assess pain, but the PAINAD has been used more widely.

Payen Behavioral Pain Scale

Critically ill intubated patients cannot self-report pain. Many of the procedures that are performed on these patients are painful. In a large multisite study with critical care patients, Thunder Project II, pain ratings for a number of patient procedures were evaluated. National results with various patient populations, from juveniles to adults, reported pain ratings for femoral line removal, turning in bed, and a number of procedures with needle sticks. Even so, a simple task such as turning a patient in bed can result in moderate intensity pain (Puntillo et al., 2001). When these patients have baseline chronic pain, the new pain the patient experiences is more significant and will result in higher intensity pain.

Assessing pain in these patients requires a tool that can detect pain behaviors, such as brow furrowing, and give an indication of pain intensity. The Payen BPS is designed specifically for critically ill intubated patients and includes a section that is designed to assess compliance with ventilation. The three assessment categories for this scale (see below) include the following:

1. Facial expression
2. Upper limb movement
3. Compliance with ventilation

To score each category, a 4-point scale is used, ranging from 1 = relaxed, no movement to 4 = grimacing, permanently retracted, and unable to control ventilation.

Payen Behavioral Pain Scale

Item	Description	Score
Facial Expression	Relaxed	1
	Partially tightened (e.g., brow lowering)	2
	Fully tightened (e.g., eyelid closing)	3
	Grimacing	4
Upper Limbs	No movement	1
	Partially bent	2
	Fully bent with finger flexion	3
	Permanently retracted	4
Compliance With Ventilation	Tolerating movement	1
	Coughing but tolerating ventilation for most of the time	2
	Fighting ventilator	3
	Unable to control ventilator	4

Source: "Assessing pain in critically ill sedated patients by using a behavioral pain scale" by J. F. Payen, O. Bru, J. L. Bosson, A. Lagrasta, E. Novel, I. Deschaux, P. Lavagne, C. Jacquot, 2001. *Critical Care Medicine, 29*(12), 1–11. Used by permission of the author.

In the original validation study, 30 critically ill intubated patients were divided into three groups based on sedation levels: mild, moderate, or heavy. Findings from the study indicate that in each group, there was a sufficient correlation with the NRS when a pain stimulus, such as a turn in bed, was performed (Payen et al., 2001). The effect of the sedation was apparent, but there was still a fair correlation with the NRS even in the group of heavily sedated patients. The tool is reliable and valid for assessing pain in this patient population. Replication studies by Aïssaoui et al. (2005) and by Purdum and D'Arcy (2006) had similar results.

Critical Care Pain Observation Tool

There are other critical care pain assessment tools, such as the Gélinas Critical Care Pain Observation Tool (CPOT), that use behavioral observation to estimate pain intensity (Gélinas, Fillion, Puntillo, Viens, & Fortier, 2006). It has four categories for assessment, facial expression, body movement, muscle tension, and compliance with the ventilator for ventilated patients or vocalization, for those critically ill patients who are extubated. The value of this tool is to provide a method of assessing both ventilated and nonventilated patients. It has proved to be both reliable and valid for assessing pain in patients who are critically ill (Gélinas et al., 2006; Gélinas & Johnston, 1997; Li, Puntillo, & Miaskowski, 2008).

Although these tools are not perfected, they do provide a means of assessing pain in patients who were once thought to be unassessable (Hutchinson et al., 2006). Because these tools are used clinically, the research support for them will develop and provide a stronger base for those tools that best fit the needs of the particular patient population.

ASSESSING PAIN IN DIFFICULT-TO-ASSESS POPULATIONS

There are some patient populations that are very difficult to assess: children, older adults, and patients with a history of substance abuse.

These patients have special needs and require special understanding when it comes to assessing pain, and there are some tools and concepts that are helpful for these groups of patients.

Assessing Pain in Older Adults

Older patients have experienced pain before. They have any number of chronic pain conditions and comorbidities that can make selecting pain medication difficult. Older patients may be reluctant to be seen as complainers and may fear adding costly medications for pain to their already crowded medication regimen (Bruckenthal & D'Arcy, 2007).

To get a good pain assessment in the older patients, make sure that any assistive devices, such as glasses and hearing aids, are in place. Convey to the patients that you have an interest in their pain and would like to help relieve the pain. Educate patients about pain assessment. Help them to understand that a good pain assessment is the best way to determine what medications and interventions could be helpful for pain relief. Include the family when it is appropriate.

Assessing Pain in Children

The two most common tools used to assess pain in children are the FACES pain scale and the face, legs, activity, cry, and consolability (FLACC) scale. The FACES scale can be used for both acute and chronic pain, whereas the FLACC is designed to be used for acute postoperative pain. The FLACC scale uses behavioral cues for assessment and has been shown to be clinically applicable for nonverbal children and those with cognitive impairment, and decreases in pain intensity scores had been demonstrated after analgesic administration (Malviya, Voepel-Lewis, Burke, Merkel, & Tait, 2006; Voepel-Lewis et al., 2008)

The FACES scale is one of the most recognized assessment tools for children. It uses six faces ranging from happy to sad, with tears on the face. To use this scale, the child is asked to pick out the face that most closely resembles how pain makes him or her feel. The FACES scale is a reliable and valid tool (Wong & DiVito-Thomas, 2006). The scale has also been used to assess pain intensity with non-Caucasian children and cognitively impaired adults (Wong & DiVito-Thomas).

Wong-Baker FACES Pain Rating Scale

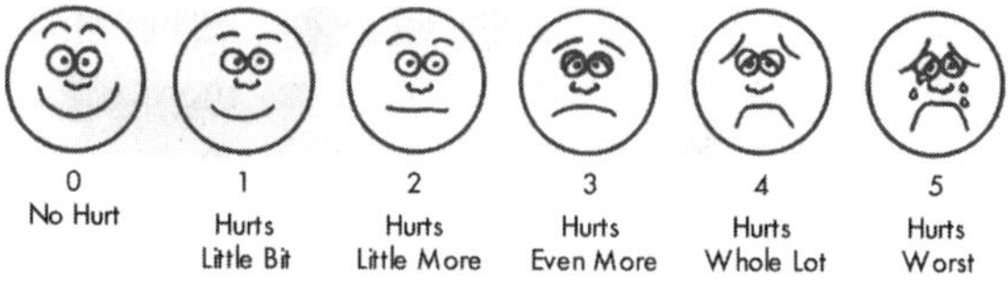

Brief word instructions: Point to each face using the words to describe the pain intensity. Ask the child to choose face that best describes own pain and record the appropriate number.

Original instructions: Explain to the person that each face is for a person who feels happy because he has no pain (hurt) or sad because he has some or a lot of pain. Face 0 is very happy because he doesn't hurt at all. Face 1 hurts just a little bit. Face 2 hurts a little more. Face 3 hurts even more. Face 4 hurts a whole lot. Face 5 hurts as much as you can imagine, although you don't have to be crying to feel this bad. Ask the person to choose the face that best desribes how he is feeling.

Rating scale is recommended for persons age 3 years and older.

From Hockenberry MJ, Wilson D: *Wong's essentials of pediatric nursing,* ed. 8, St. Louis, 2009, Mosby. Used with permission. Copyright Mosby.

FLACC Behavioral Scale

Categories	Scoring 0	1	2
Face	No particular expression or smile	Occasional grimace or frown, withdrawn, disinterested	Frequent to constant frown, clenched jaw, quivering chin
Legs	Normal position or relaxed	Uneasy, restless, tense	Kicking, or legs drawn up

(Continued)

(Continued)

Activity	Lying quietly, normal position, moves easily	Squirming, shifting back and forth, tense	Arched, rigid, or jerking
Cry	No cry (awake or asleep)	Moans or whimpers, occasional complaint	Crying steadily, screams or sobs, frequent complaints
Consolability	Content, relaxed	Reassured by occasional touching, hugging, or being talked to, distractable	Difficult to console or comfort

Each of the five categories (F) Face; (L) Legs; (A) Activity; (C) Cry; (C) Consolability is scored from 0-2, which results in a total score between zero and ten.

Assessing Pain in Patients With a Substance Abuse History

Illicit substance abuse and prescription drug abuse and misuse has been steadily increasing at an alarming rate. Patients who have a history of substance abuse are difficult to assess for pain as they often will report continued levels of high-intensity pain despite efforts to control the pain.

It can be very frustrating for a nurse to give large doses of pain medication to these patients and have the patient continue to report high-intensity pain. Some of this response is related to alterations in the patient's physiology that are created with continued use of opioid medications or illicit substances and causes the patient's body to become more sensitive to pain. This heightened sensitivity to pain is called *opioid-induced hyperalgesia*, and it can occur as soon as 1 month after opioid use/abuse begins (Chu et al., 2006). It would then be expected that these patients would report higher pain levels and require more pain medication to control their pain.

To perform a pain assessment in a patient who is actively using illicit substances or has a history of substance abuse, it is important to remember the following:

- A nonjudgmental approach is best. To get accurate information, the patient should feel that he or she can trust you with the information, and that he or she will not be judged.
- Determine when the patient last used an illicit substance.
- Determine what the substance is and how much the patient uses every day.
- Assess for any cosubstance abuse, such as combinations of alcohol, heroin, marijuana, cocaine, and so forth.
- Reassure the patient that you need this information to help determine what types of medication or interventions will help to control the pain.
- Reassess the patient's pain at regular intervals to determine if the pain medication has been effective in reducing pain.
- Remember that these patients may have had bad experiences with other health care providers, and try to gain trust so that they feel comfortable talking to you about their pain. (More information on treating patients with chronic pain and substance abuse will be provided later in the book in Section V.)

BARRIERS TO PAIN ASSESSMENT

There are some barriers that make accurate pain assessment difficult for nurses.

- Bias
- Cultural influences
- Family values
- Belief systems (Harrison, 1991)

Nurses still have difficulty accepting the patient's report of pain as valid and credible (Berry et al., 2006; D'Arcy, 2008; Donovan et al., 1987; Drayer et al., 1999; Grossman et al., 1991; Paice et al., 1991). To minimize the effects of these factors on pain assessment, it is important for the nurse to recognize these factors and consciously work to derive a pain assessment that is as accurate as possible.

Today's health care providers are being held accountable for the quality of their pain management, including assessment. It is incumbent on each nurse who performs a pain assessment to attempt to get a pain assessment as accurate as possible. When pain assessment is poorly done, it can affect the patient's plan of care and adversely impact outcomes.

Focusing on pain relief as the primary end to the assessment process and treatment selection will help control fears and biases that can negatively affect patient care. Accepting and believing the patient's report of pain is essential to performing a good pain assessment.

Using a recognized, reliable, and valid pain assessment tool; believing the patient; and accepting the patient's report of pain in a nonjudgmental fashion will provide the patient with the best chance for adequate pain relief.

Case Study

Mrs. Swanson, 85 years old, is admitted from the local nursing home with what appears to be abdominal pain. She has not been eating for 2 days, has not had a bowel movement in 3 days, and her abdomen is distended and firm. When you try to assess her pain, you notice that she is moaning and pushes your hand away when you try to gently palpate her abdomen. As she waits in the emergency department, she has a cardiac arrest, is coded successfully, and is intubated and transferred to the critical care unit. Her diagnosis is perforated ulcer and she is at high risk for peritonitis and has been scheduled for emergency surgery.

Questions to Consider

1. You know Mrs. Swanson had pain behaviors when she was admitted. How will you assess her pain?
2. Would you say her pain is severe or a lower intensity pain?
3. What tools are suggested for assessing pain in the critical care unit?
4. What pain tools could be used for Mrs. Swanson during her hospitalization?

REFERENCES

Aïssaoui, Y., Zeggwagh, A. A., Zekraoui, A., Abidi, K., & Abouqal, R. (2005). Validation of a behavioral pain scale in critically ill, sedated, and mechanically ventilated patients. *Anesthesia and Analgesia, 101*(5), 1470–1476.

American Geriatrics Society. (2002). The management of persistent pain in older persons—The American Geriatrics Society Panel on Persistent Pain in Older Persons. *Journal of the American Geriatrics Society, 50*(6), S205–S224.

Berry, P. H., Covington, E., Dahl, J., Katz, J., & Miaskowski, C. (2006). *Pain: Current understanding of assessment, management, and treatments.* Reston, VA: National Pharmaceutical Council, Inc. and The Joint Commission on Accreditation of Healthcare Organizations.

Bruckenthal, P., & D'Arcy, Y. (2007). Assessment and management of pain in older persons: A review of the basics. *Topics in Advanced Practice ejournal, 2007*(1). Retrieved September 17, 2009, from http://www.medscape.com/viewarticle/55638

Chok, B. (1998). An overview of the visual analogue scale and the McGill pain questionnaire. *Physiotherapy Singapore, 1*(3), 88–93.

Chu, L. F., Clark, D. J., & Angst, M. S. (2006). Opioid tolerance and hyperalgesia in chronic pain patients after one month of oral morphine therapy: A preliminary prospective study. *The Journal of Pain, 7*(1), 43–48.

D'Arcy, Y. (2007). *Pain management: Evidence-based tools and techniques for nursing professionals.* Marblehead, MA: HCPro.

D'Arcy, Y. (2008). Be in the know about pain management. *The Nurse Practitioner, 38*(6), 43–49.

Daut, R. L., Cleeland, C. S., & Flanery, R. (1983). Development of the Wisconsin Brief Pain Questionnaire to assess pain in cancer or other diseases. *Pain, 17*(2), 197–210.

Donovan, M., Dillon, P., & McGuire, L. (1987). Incidence and characteristics of pain in a sample of medical-surgical inpatients. *Pain, 30*(1), 69–78.

Drayer, R. A., Henderson, J., & Reidenberg, M. (1999). Barriers to better pain control in hospitalized patients. *Journal of Pain & Symptom Management, 17*(6), 434–440.

Dworkin, R. H., Turk, D. C., Revicki, D. A., Harding, G., Coyne, K. S., & Peirce-Sandner, S., . . . Melzack, R. (2009). Development and initial validation of an expanded and revised version of the short-form McGill pain Questionnaire (SF-MPQ-2). *Pain, 144*(1–2), 35–42.

Feldt, K. S. (2000). The Checklist of Non-verbal Pain Indicators (CNPI). *Pain Management Nursing, 1*(1), 13–21.

Feldt, K. S., Ryden, M. B., & Miles, S. (1998). Treatment of pain in cognitively impaired compared with cognitively intact older patients with hip fractures. *Journal of the American Geriatrics Society, 46*(9), 1079–1085.

Gélinas, C., Fillion, L., Puntillo, K., Viens, C., & Fortier, M. (2006). Validation of the critical-care pain observation tool in adult patients. *American Journal of Critical Care, 15*(4), 420–427.

Gélinas, C., & Johnston, M. (1997). Pain assessment in the critically ill ventilated adult: Validation of the critical-care pain observation tool and physiologic indicators. *Clinical Journal of Pain, 23*(6), 497–505.

Ger, L. P., Ho, S. T., Sun, W. Z., Wang, M. S., & Cleeland, C. S. (1999). Validation of the brief pain inventory in a Taiwanese population. *Journal of Pain and Symptom Management, 18*(5), 316–322.

Gracely, R. H., & Dubner, R. (1987). Reliability of verbal descriptor scales of painfulness. *Pain, 29*(2), 175–185.

Graham, C., Bond, S. S., Gerkovich, M. M., & Cook, M. R. (1980). Use of the McGill Pain Questionnaire in the assessment of cancer pain: Replicability and consistency. *Pain, 8*(3), 377–387.

Grossman, S. A., Sheidler, V. R., Swedeen, K., Mucenski, J., & Piantadosi, S. (1991). Correlation of patient and caregiver ratings of cancer pain. *Journal of Pain and Symptom Management, 6*(2), 53–57.

Harrison, A. (1991). Assessing patients' pain: Identifying reasons for error. *Journal of Advanced Nursing, 16,* 1018–1025.

Herr, K., Bjoro, K., & Decker, S. (2006). Tools for assessment of pain in nonverbal older adults with dementia: A state-of-the-science review. *Journal of Pain and Symptom Management, 31*(2), 170–192.

Herr, K., Coyne, P., Key, T., Manworren, R., McCaffery, M., Merkel, S., . . . Wild, L. (2006). Pain assessment in the nonverbal patient: Position statement with clinical practice recommendations. *Pain Management Nursing, 7*(2), 44–52.

Hutchison, R. W., Tucker, W. F., Jr., Kim, S., & Gilder, R. (2006). Evaluation of a behavioral assessment tool for the individual unable to self-report pain. *American Journal of Hospice and Palliative Care, 23*(4), 328–331.

Klepstad, P., Loge, J. H., Borchgervink, P. C., Mendoza, T. R., Cleeland, C., & Kaasa, S. (2002). The Norwegian Brief Pain Inventory Questionnaire: Translation and validation in cancer pain patients. *Journal of Pain and Symptom Management, 24*(5), 517–525.

Lane, P., Kuntupis, M., MacDonald, S., McCarthy, P., Panke, J. A., Warden, V., & Volicer, L. (2003). A pain assessment tool for people with advanced Alzheimer's and other progressive dementias. *Home Healthcare Nurse, 21*(1), 32–37.

Li, D., Puntillo, K., & Miaskowski, C. (2008). A review of objective pain measures for use with critical care adult patients unable to self report. *Journal of Pain, 9*(1), 2–10.

Malviya, S., Voepel-Lewis, T., Burke, C., Merkel, S., & Tait, A. R. (2006). The revised FLACC observational pain tool: Improved reliability and validity for pain assessment in children with cognitive impairment. *Pediatric Anesthesiology, 16*(3), 258–265.

McDonald, D. D., & Weiskopf, C. S. A. (2001). Adult patients' postoperative pain descriptions and responses to the short-form McGill Pain Questionnaire. *Clinical Nursing Research, 10*(4), 442–452.

McIntyre, D. L., Hopkins, P. M., & Harris, S. R. (1995). Evaluation of pain and functional activity in patellofemoral pain syndrome: Reliability and validity of two assessment tools. *Physiotherapy of Canada, 47*(3), 164–170.

Melzack, R. (1975). The McGill Pain Questionnaire: Major properties and scoring methods. *Pain, 1*(3), 277–299.

Melzack, R. (1987). The short-form McGill Pain Questionnaire. *Pain, 30*(2), 191–197.

Merkel, S., Voepel-Lewis, T., Shayevitz, J., & Malviya, S. (1997). The FLACC: A behavioral scale for scoring postoperative pain in young children. *Pediatric Nursing, 23*(3), 293– 297.

Mystakidou, K., Mendoza, T, Tsilika, E., Befon, S., Parpa, G., Bellos, G., . . . Cleeland, C. (2001). Greek Brief Pain Inventory: Validation and utility in cancer pain. *Oncology, 60*(1), 35–42.

Mystakidou, K., Parpa, E., Tsilika, E., Kaladopoulou, O., Georgaki, S., Galanos, A., & Vlahos, L. (2002). Greek McGill Pain Questionnaire: Validation and utility in cancer patients. *Journal of Pain and Symptom Management, 24*(4), 379–387.

Paice, J. A., Mahon, S. M., & Faut-Callahan, M. (1991). Factors associated with adequate pain control in hospitalized postsurgical patients diagnosed with cancer. *Cancer Nursing, 14*(6), 298–305.

Payen, J. F., Bru, O., Bosson, J. L., Lagrasta, A., Novel, E., Deschaux, I., . . . Jacquot, C. (2001). Assessing pain in critically ill sedated patients by using a behavioral pain scale. *Critical Care Medicine, 29*(12), 2258–2263.

Puntillo, K. A., White, C., Morris, A. B., Perdue, S. T., Stanik-Hutt, J., Thompson, C. L., & Wild, L. R. (2001). Patients' perceptions and responses to procedural pain: Results from the Thunder Project II. *American Journal of Critical Care, 10*(4), 238–251.

Purdum, A., & D'Arcy, Y. (2006). *A comparison of two behavioral pain scales in intubated intensive care unit (ICU) patients.* San Antonio, TX: American Pain Society.

Radbruch, L., Loick, G., Kiencke, P., Lindena, G., Sabatowski, R., Grond, S., . . . Cleeland, C. S. (1999). Validation of the German version of the Brief Pain Inventory. *Journal of Pain & Symptom Management, 18*(3), 180–187.

Raichle, K. A., Osborne, T. L., Jensen, M. P., & Cardenas, D. (2006). The reliability and validity of pain interference measures in persons with spinal cord injury. *Journal of Pain, 7*(3), 179–186.

Tan, G., Jensen, M. P., Thornby, J. I., & Shanti, B. F. (2004). Validation of the Brief Pain Inventory for chronic nonmalignant pain. *Journal of Pain & Symptom Management, 5*(2), 133–137.

Tittle, M. B., McMillan, S. C., & Hagan, S. (2003). Validating the Brief Pain Inventory for use with surgical patients with cancer. *Oncology Nursing Forum, 30*(2), 325–330.

Warden, V., Hurley, A. C., & Volicer, L. (2003). Development and psychometric evaluation of the Pain Assessment in Advanced Dementia (PAINAD) Scale. *Journal of the American Medical Directors Association, 4*(1), 9–15.

Wilkie, D. J., Savedra, M. C., Holzemer, W. L., Tesler, M. D., & Paul, S. M. (1990). Use of the McGill Pain Questionnaire to measure pain: A meta-analysis. *Nursing Research, 39*(1), 36–41.

Williams, V. S. L., Smith, M. Y., & Fehnel, S. E. (2006). The validity and utility of the BPI interference measures for evaluating the impact of osteoarthritic pain. *Journal of Pain & Symptom Management, 31*(1), 48–57.

Voepel-Lewis, T., Malviya, S., Tait, A. R., Merkel, S., Foster, R., Krane, E. J., & Davis, P. J. (2008). A comparison of the clinical utility of pain assessment tools for children with cognitive impairment. *Anesthesia and Analgesia, 106*(1), 72–78.

Wong, D., & DiVito-Thomas, P. (2006). *The validity, reliability, and preference of the Wong-Baker FACES Pain Rating Scale among Chinese, Japanese, and Thai children.* Retrieved from www.mosbysdrugconsult.com/WOW/op080.html

III

Medications and Treatments for Acute Pain

6

Medication Management With Nonopioid Medications

OVERVIEW OF MEDICATION MANAGEMENT

The mainstay for treating acute pain is medication management. Most patients with a pain complaint expect to receive a medication prescription when they see their health care provider. However, for some conditions, such as acute low back pain, the current recommendations are acetaminophen/nonsteroidal anti-inflammatory drugs (NSAIDs) and continued activity rather than opioids and bedrest (Chou et al., 2009). About 15% of the patients who have acute low back pain progress to chronic low back pain. Medication management for chronic low back pain is recommended, accompanied by a plan of care that includes medications along with other therapies, such as physical therapy and counseling (D'Arcy, 2009c). Opioids currently are, in most cases, reserved for severe pain that impairs functionality (Chou et al., 2009).

To treat acute pain with medications requires a pain assessment; history and physical examination; and a medication review that includes over-the-counter medications, herbal supplements, and vitamins (Bruckenthal, 2007). Most patients with pain try to self-treat first and have tried pain medications in the past and know which work the best and which are less effective. When patients have information about medications that are effective for relieving their pain, consider this to be information that is similar to what a patient with diabetes provides about his or her daily insulin doses to a new health care provider. Just because a patient is familiar with medication names and doses does not make him or her a "drug seeker."

There are genetic factors that influence the effectiveness of pain medications in a specific individual, so when a patient says, "the only medication that works for me is morphine," it may really be a reflection of how his or her genetic makeup has reacted to medications tried in the past. The patient should never be penalized or negatively labeled for providing information on how specific medications have worked for him or her in the past.

This section of the book will provide information about using pain medications of various types, NSAIDs, opioids, and other coanalgesics, such as antidepressants. The information will be taken from current guidelines developed by the American Pain Society (APS), the American Geriatrics Society (AGS), the American Academy of Pain Medicine (AAPM), and other national organizations. Included will be an order set for pain management based on the World Health Organization (WHO) analgesic ladder and medication charts (Figure 6.1). The topics of addiction, dependency, and tolerance will be discussed in the last section of the book. Information on integrative therapies that can be combined with medication management will be provided at the end of this section.

GENERAL GUIDELINES

All patients have the right to have their pain treated, and most health care providers make honest efforts at getting the patient's pain to a tolerable level (Brennan, Carr, & Cousins, 2007). Most chronic patients with acute or surgical pain realize that "pain free" is not a reasonable goal to set and that a risk-benefit analysis is used to determine what type of medication management will provide the best outcome for the patient. However, pain has become an extremely common patient complaint that many times requires the use of nonopioid medications, opioid analgesics, and coanalgesics.

Most prescribers have very little concern when opioids are needed for short-term pain management, but when opioid therapy is

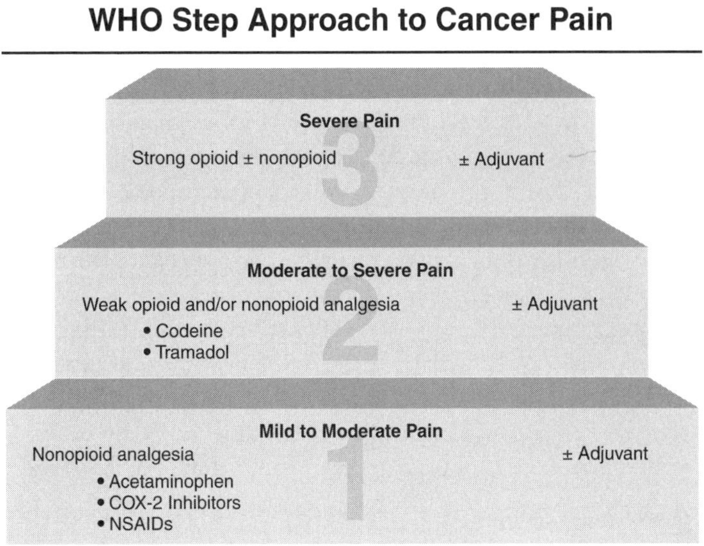

Figure 6.1 ■ Analgesic ladder

required for the long term, their concern increases, and fears of addicting the patient to the medication or fear of increased regulatory oversight can affect the prescriber's willingness to continue providing opioid medications to the patient with chronic pain (D'Arcy, 2009a). For acute pain, this issue is not as significant, but there are still some health care providers who feel that they are contributing to addiction when opioids are used in the acute care setting. This can lead the prescriber to consider the nonopioid medications as a first-line medication when an opioid may be indicated. Alternatively, the prescriber may try an opioid that he or she perceives has a lower potential for abuse or addiction, such as acetaminophen with codeine, even though the patient may be reporting severe pain. Selecting a medication that will be effective for the patient's pain complaint can be by trial and error until the right medication and dose are found.

Some patients who have acute pain will progress to chronic pain management. All patients who are being considered for chronic opioid therapy should be screened for risks that include opioid misuse, development of aberrant medication-taking behaviors, and addiction (Chou et al., 2009). The development of a comprehensive treatment plan that includes the use of various medications is extremely important to the success of pain management (Institute for Clinical Systems Improvement, 2008). If long-term opioids are being considered, an opioid agreement may be created that outlines when the medications will be refilled, the risks and benefits of the medications, the use of random urine screens, and the consequences of violating the agreement (Trescot et al., 2008). A sample opioid agreement can be obtained at the website of the AAPM. At the other end of the spectrum, the undertreatment of pain can produce a plethora of unwanted side effects, especially with older patients. Some of the significant consequences of undertreated pain include the following:

- Depression
- Impaired cognition
- Sleep disturbances
- Poorer clinical outcome
- Decreased functional ability
- Decreased quality of life
- Anxiety
- Decreased socialization
- Increased health care utilization and costs (AGS, 2002; Brennan et al., 2007; D'Arcy, 2007; Karani, 2004)

In a recent survey conducted by Stanford University, 40% of the respondents reported that pain interfered with enjoyment of life and pleasurable activities and that chronic pain adversely affected their mood (Stanos, Fishbain, & Fishman, 2009). Although 63% of the survey respondents indicated that they had gone to their health care provider, only 31% of the patients reported that they had either complete or a great deal of pain relief. In addition, less than 50% reported a lot of control over their pain. What this tells us about acute pain that progresses to chronic pain and its management is that the problem is very big and the ability of health care providers to control the pain is limited.

Among pain specialists, there is currently a movement toward considering chronic pain as a disease in and of itself (Brennan et al., 2007). There is also evidence to support the idea that untreated or undertreated acute pain can lead to more difficult-to-treat chronic pain syndromes, such as complex regional pain syndromes. Becoming more aware of patients with acute pain who report high levels of pain for many clinic visits or return visits is important for providers working with these patients, because this can be the beginning of a chronic pain condition. The effect of chronic pain on the patient is so profound that it constitutes a major threat to health and wellness. Unrelieved chronic pain can have many different physiologic effects, such as the following:

- Reduced mobility
- Loss of strength
- Disturbed sleep
- Decreased immune function
- Increased susceptibility to disease
- Dependence on medications for pain relief
- Depression and anxiety (Brennan et al., 2007)

Because of the magnitude of the problem of pain and the impact on the individual patient's well-being, health care providers need to become proficient in prescribing and dosing medications for pain of all types. The WHO developed an analgesic ladder that can provide guidance to prescribers about their choices of pain medications. Although the ladder was originally developed for cancer pain, it has been adapted for use in many areas of pain management to include acute pain.

Level I Medications—Mild to Moderate Pain

Medications to treat mild to moderate pain, which are on the first step of the ladder, include acetaminophen; NSAIDs, both selective and nonselective; and adjuvant medications or coanalgesics. These medications can add to pain relief, although they are not primarily classed as pain medications. These medications include antidepressants, anticonvulsants, muscle relaxants, and topical medications.

Level II Medications—Moderate to Severe Pain

On the middle step of the ladder are the moderate to severe pain medications, for example a combination medication with an opioid, such as hydrocodone or oxycodone (OxyContin), and acetaminophen. In addition, tramadol (Ultram) and tapentadol (Nucynta), medications with combined mu agonist and selective serotonin reuptake inhibitor actions, are included in this level of medications for moderate pain. Adjuvant medications for this level could include the muscle relaxants and antidepressants of the lower level, but the acetaminophen or NSAIDs of the lower level could also be used at this point for additional pain relief.

Level III Medications—Severe Pain

Patients who are reporting severe pain require strong opioid medications for pain relief. Included in this group of medications are the opioids, such as morphine, fentanyl (Sublimaze), hydromorphone (Dilaudid), and methadone (Dolophine). As with the other steps, adjuvant medication should be continued here to help reduce opioid needs and provide additional pain relief (adapted from D'Arcy, 2007).

Clinical Pearl

Although the WHO analgesic ladder provides some guidance in the choice of medications, the overall assessment, history and physical comorbidities, and organ functions need to be considered when selecting a medication for pain.

It is important to remember that the patient's report of pain is more than a number. There are many pieces of the patient puzzle that need to fit together just right to find an effective method for pain relief. Although the severity ratings of the analgesic ladder are a guide to choosing the correct medication because there is a group of medications in each level, the practitioners can individualize the medication selection. The efficacy of the medication is an individualized response based on the patient's report of decreased pain or increased functionality (D'Arcy, 2007).

PHYSICIAN'S ORDERS
Pain Management Standard Order Set

ALLERGIES ➤

I HEREBY AUTHORIZE THE PHARMACY TO DISPENSE A GENERIC EQUIVALENT UNLESS THE PARTICULAR DRUG IS CIRCLED.

PATIENT PLATE

ORDERS ***PLEASE WRITE WITH BALLPOINT PEN***

Medications must be written with one dose and one time interval. Select only one medication from each section.

Mild Pain. Pain Intensity Rating 1-3
☐ Tylenol ☐ Tylenol #3 (Tylenol with codeine)
*No more than 4 grams of Tylenol per day
☐ Ibuprofen (starting dose 200 mgs twice a day)
☐ Celebrex (Starting dose 100 mg twice a day - no more than 400 mgs per day)
☐ PO ☐ PRN ☐ Scheduled
Dose ☐ One tablet ☐ Two tablets ☐ Other ______
Interval-every ☐ 4 hours ☐ 6 hours ☐ 8 hours

Moderate Pain. Pain Intensity Rating 4-6 * Consider total daily intake of Tylenol
☐ Vicodin (Hydrocodone with Tylenol) ☐ Percocet (Oxycodone with Tylenol)
☐ Oxy IR (oxycodone) ☐ Oxycontin (extended release oxycodone)
*Suggested starting dose one tablet every 4 hours except for oxycontin which is given every 12 hours
☐ PO ☐ PRN ☐ Scheduled
Dose ☐ One tablet ☐ Two tablets ☐ Other ______
Interval-every ☐ 4 hours ☐ 6 hours ☐ 8 hours ☐ 12 hours

Severe Pain. Pain Intensity Rating 7-10
☐ MSIR (oral morphine) ☐ MS Contin (Extended release morphine)
Suggested starting dose 15 milligrams every 4 hours except MS Contin which is given every 12 hours
☐ Dilaudid (hydromorphone) Suggested starting dose 2 milligrams every 4 hours
☐ PO ☐ PRN ☐ Scheduled
Dose ______
Interval-every ☐ 4 hours ☐ 6 hours ☐ 8 hours ☐ 12 hours

Parenteral Pain Medications- For use as primary medication or for breakthrough pain
☐ Morphine (suggested 2 milligrams every hour) ☐ Dilaudid (suggested- 0.5 milligrams every 3 hours)
*Caution in elderly. May accumulate with decreased renal clearance
☐ Fentanyl - dosed in **MICROGRAMS** (suggested 25 **micrograms** every hour)
☐ Toradol * Five day maximum use * reduce dose in elderly * Creat > 1.2 or hx of GI bleed-do not use suggested 15 milligrams every 6 hours
☐ IV ☐ SQ ☐ IM ☐ PRN ☐ Scheduled
Dose ______
Interval-every ☐ hour ☐ 2 hours ☐ 4 hours ☐ 6 hours ☐ 8 hours ☐ 12 hours

Fentanyl Patch
☐ Duragesic patch - not recommended for acute postoperative use, change every 72 hours
Start opioid naïve patients on 25 **microgram** patch. Takes 12 - 18 hours to begin relieving pain.
☐ 25 microgram ☐ 50 microgram ☐ 75 microgram ☐ 100 microgram ☐ 200 microgram

Laxative
☐ Senakot one tab ☐ Milk of Magnesia 30 ml ☐ Dulcolax one tab/Suppository ☐ Colace 100 mg
☐ Other ______
☐ PO ☐ Rectal suppository ☐ PRN ☐ Scheduled
☐ every day ☐ twice per day

Antiemetic
☐ Phenergan ☐ Reglan ☐ Zofran ☐ Compazine ☐ Scopolamine patch 1.5 mg disk - change every 3 days
☐ PO ☐ Rectal ☐ IV ☐ PRN ☐ Scheduled
Dose ______
Interval-every ☐ 4 hours ☐ 6 hours ☐ 8 hours ☐ 12 hours

PAIN DISTRESS/ INTENSITY SCALE

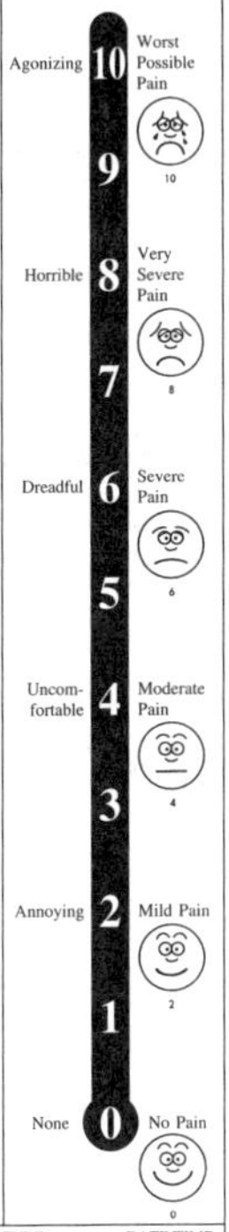

PLEASE WRITE WITH BALLPOINT PEN	UNIT SECRETARY	DATE/TIME	RN SIGNATURE	DATE/TIME	PHYSICIAN'S SIGNATURE	DATE/TIME

MEDICAL RECORDS

Figure 6.2 ■ Pain management order set exemplar. *Source:* Courtesy of Suburban Hospital–Johns Hopkins Medicine, Bethesda, MD.

For treating acute pain, a pain management order set that clarifies which medications are available to treat the stated level of pain is useful for general directions. A sample of an order set is included in this chapter (Figure 6.2). Another use for this order set is education.

It can help prescribers understand which medication is appropriate to treat the various levels of pain. This avoids the use of acetaminophen with codeine to treat severe pain and indicates which medications might be better choices.

NONOPIOID ANALGESICS FOR PAIN (ACETAMINOPHEN AND NSAIDs)

Although acetaminophen and NSAIDs are considered to be weaker medications for pain, they can provide a good baseline of relief that can help decrease the amount of opioid required to treat pain. Both acetaminophen and NSAIDs are seriously overlooked and underutilized as coanalgesics when higher intensity pain is reported. Multimodal analgesia, which is recommended for complex pain needs and for postoperative pain relief, may consist of any combination of medications that may include the use of acetaminophen and NSAIDs. However, there are some important considerations when adding these medications into a pain regimen. These medications are not benign and have risk potential that should be considered prior to use in all patients. They also have maximum dose levels that create a ceiling for dose escalations.

■ *Acetaminophen (APAP, Paracetamol)*

Acetaminophen is used worldwide to treat pain. Known as paracetamol in Europe, it is associated with the Tylenol brand in the United States and is widely added to many over-the-counter pain relievers, such as Excedrin, Midol, and the various Tylenol products. It is available as tablets, gel caps, and elixirs, and as pediatric formulations. Most home medicine chests have some type of acetaminophen compound that the family uses for relief of minor aches and pains. Because it is so popular and easy to obtain, some 24.6 billion doses were sold in 2008 (Pan, 2009).

Acetaminophen is classed as a para-acetaminophen derivative (*Nursing 2010 Drug Handbook*, 2009), and it has a similar pain relief profile to aspirin without the potential to damage the gastric mucosa (APS, 2008). Pain relief efficacy of acetaminophen is superior to placebo but slightly less effective than NSAIDs (APS, 2008). The action of the medication is thought to be the inhibition of prostaglandins and other pain-producing substances (*Nursing 2010 Drug Handbook*, 2009). It is entirely metabolized in the liver and can cause blood pressure elevations (Buvanendran & Lipman, 2009).

Advantages of acetaminophen over NSAIDs include the following:

- Fewer gastrointestinal (GI) adverse effects
- Fewer GI complications

In general, acetaminophen is safe and effective when used according to the directions and labeling on over-the-counter preparations and any prescription-strength medication information. There are serious concerns today about acetaminophen overdose, both intentional and unintentional. The U.S. Food and Drug Administration (FDA) has been holding hearings and is considering reducing the recommendations for the daily total dose from 4,000 mg per day to a lower limit. The FDA is also considering making the 500-mg strength tablets available only by prescription and limiting the number of doses in each package (Alazraki, 2009).

The concerns underlying these fears are related to some very serious statistics about the increase in liver disease related to acetaminophen use. There is a clear connection with acetaminophen overuse and liver disease and failure. Total acetaminophen doses should not exceed 4,000 mg per day, including any combination medication taken by the patient that may include acetaminophen (Trescott, Helm, Hansen, et al., 2008). Even at this dose, there is an associated risk of hepatotoxicity (APS, 2008).

From 1998 to 2003, acetaminophen was the leading cause of acute liver failure in the United States (Alazraki, 2009). Between 1990 and 1998, there were 56,000 emergency department visits, 26,000 hospitalizations, and 458 deaths reportedly connected to acetaminophen overdoses (Alazraki, 2009). Many of these overdoses were unintentional and caused by a knowledge deficit about the "hidden" acetaminophen found in combination medications. Some of the most common prescription strength combinations with acetaminophen include the following:

- Tylenol #3
- Vicodin
- Percocet
- Ultracet

Other over-the-counter medications that can contain hidden acetaminophen include the following:

- Alka-Seltzer Plus
- Cough syrups, such as NightQuil/DayQuil cold and flu relief
- Over-the-counter pain relievers, such as Pamprin and Midol maximum-strength menstrual formula

Care should be taken with older patients, patients with liver-impaired function, and any patient who uses alcohol regularly (AGS, 2009; APS, 2008). In these cases, acetaminophen doses should not exceed 2,000 mg per day or it should not be used at all (AGS, 2009). The risk of liver failure is very real. It is imperative for all patients who are taking Tylenol to read and understand the medication administration guidelines and recommendations. Exceeding daily recommended doses of acetaminophen can have deadly consequences.

One little-known impact is the effect of acetaminophen on the anticoagulant warfarin (Coumadin). Careful monitoring of anticoagulation should take place when a patient is taking both acetaminophen and warfarin because acetaminophen is an underrecognized cause of over-anticoagulation when both medications are being used concomitantly (APS, 2008).

■ *Aspirin*

Aspirin is one of the oldest pain relievers known to humans. It is classed as a salicylate. Before the beginning of modern medicine, salicylate-rich willow bark was used as one of the earliest forms of pain relief. Many Americans use aspirin for minor aches and pains, and because of its action on platelet activity, it has been promoted for early in-the-field treatment for patients who are experiencing heart attack. It was traditionally used for pain relief of osteoarthritis, rheumatoid arthritis, and for other inflammatory conditions but has been replaced by newer NSAIDs (APS, 2008; *Nursing 2010 Drug Handbook*, 2009).

Aspirin is available in many different doses, but the most common dose is 500 to 1,000 mg every 4 or 6 hours with a maximum dose of 4,000 mg per day (APS, 2008). It is available in buffered, sustained-release, and chewable formulations.

Despite its easy availability and widespread use, there are some serious adverse events connected with regular aspirin use. These include the following:

- GI distress
- GI ulceration and bleeding
- Prolonged bleeding times
- Reye syndrome
- Aspirin hypersensitivity

These reactions to aspirin are quite serious and, in some cases, life threatening. GI ulceration and bleeding can cause death. Aspirin is not recommended for children younger than the age of 12 because of the potential for Reye syndrome, which can develop when a child has a viral illness and aspirin is given for pain relief (APS, 2008). Aspirin hypersensitivity reactions can be minor or very severe. A minor reaction presents as a respiratory reaction with rhinitis, asthma, or nasal polyps. A smaller group of patients can get more serious reactions that include the following:

- Urticaria
- Wheals
- Angioneurotic edema
- Hypotension
- Shock and syncope (APS, 2008)

Although aspirin seems like a very simple analgesic, care should be taken with any aspirin use.

THE NSAID DEBATE

NSAIDs of all types are commonly used for pain that is mild to moderate in intensity. They can be used for pain that is inflammatory and as an analgesic for low-level pain or as a coanalgesic. They are available in different combinations in both prescription strength and over-the-counter preparations. They do have a maximum dose that limits dose escalation beyond the maximum dose ceiling.

NSAIDs have two different types of actions: selective and nonselective.

- *Nonselective NSAIDs* affect all types of prostaglandins found in the stomach, kidneys, heart, and other organs of the body.
- *Selective NSAIDs* protect the prostaglandins that coat the stomach lining but do affect the other types of prostaglandins found elsewhere in the body.

The most common use of NSAIDs is to treat pain that is caused by inflammation, such as arthritis or common musculoskeletal injuries (APS, 2008; D'Arcy, 2007).

NSAIDs have long been a standard for pain relief in older patients. Relatively cheap, they are easily accessible at most supermarkets or drugstores. They are available as over-the-counter formulations and in prescription strength as well. The most common uses are for arthritis pain, headaches, and minor sprains and strains.

Based on the differences in actions, the NSAIDs are clearly divided into two classes: *nonselective* and *COX-2 selective*. The nonselective NSAIDs include ibuprofen (Motrin, Advil), naproxen (Naprosyn), and ketoprofen (Orudis). They affect production of the prostaglandins that coat and protect the lining of the stomach and those that are found in other organs of the body, including the kidneys and the heart. The only COX-2 selective NSAID medication available at this time is celecoxib (Celebrex). Celecoxib spares the stomach prostaglandins and does not affect platelet aggregation, so blood clotting is not affected. Mechanisms for both types of NSAIDs can be found at http://www.fda.gov.

Newer research from the FDA indicates that all NSAIDs, not only the COX-2 selective medications such as Celebrex, have the potential for increased cardiovascular risk, renovascular risk, stroke, and myocardial infarction (Bennett, Daugherty, Herrington, et al., 2005; D'Arcy, 2007). GI bleeding with NSAIDs continues to be a risk; for those patients who are taking aspirin as a cardiac prophylaxis, the risk increases severalfold with concomitant NSAID and aspirin use (D'Arcy, 2007) (Exhibit 6.1).

Exhibit 6.1

Medication Guide for Non-Steroidal Anti-Inflammatory Drugs (NSAIDs.)
(See the end of this Medication Guide for a list of prescription NSAID medicines.)

What is the most important information I should know about medicines called Non-Steroidal Anti-Inflammatory Drugs (NSAIDs)?

NSAID medicines may increase the chance of a heart attack or stroke that can lead to death. This chance increases:
- with longer use of NSAID medicines
- in people who have heart disease

NSAID medicines should never be used right before or after a heart surgery called a "coronary artery bypass graft (CABG)."

NSAID medicines can cause ulcers and bleeding in the stomach and intestines at any time during treatment. Ulcers and bleeding:
- can happen without warning symptoms
- may cause death

The chance of a person getting an ulcer or bleeding increases with:
- taking medicines called "corticosteroids" and "anticoagulants"
- longer use
- smoking
- drinking alcohol
- older age
- having poor health

NSAID medicines should only be used:
- exactly as prescribed
- at the lowest dose possible for your treatment
- for the shortest time needed

What are Non-Steroidal Anti-Inflammatory Drugs (NSAIDs)?
NSAID medicines are used to treat pain and redness, swelling, and heat (inflammation) from medical conditions such as:
- different types of arthritis
- menstrual cramps and other types of short-term pain

Who should not take a Non-Steroidal Anti-Inflammatory Drug (NSAID)?
Do not take an NSAID medicine:
- if you had an asthma attack, hives, or other allergic reaction with aspirin or any other NSAID medicine
- for pain right before or after heart bypass surgery

Tell your healthcare provider:
- about all of your medical conditions.
- about all of the medicines you take. NSAIDs and some other medicines can interact with each other and cause serious side effects. **Keep a list of your medicines to show to your healthcare provider and pharmacist.**
- if you are pregnant. **NSAID medicines should not be used by pregnant women late in their pregnancy.**
- if you are breastfeeding. **Talk to your doctor.**

What are the possible side effects of Non-Steroidal Antl-Inflammatory Drugs (NSAIDs)?

Serious side effects include:
- heart attack
- stroke
- high blood pressure
- heart failure from body swelling (fluid retention)
- kidney problems including kidney failure
- bleeding and ulcers in the stomach and intestine
- low red blood cells (anemia)
- life-threatening skin reactions
- life-threatening allergic reactions
- liver problems including liver failure
- asthma attacks in people who have asthma

Other side effects include:
- stomach pain
- constipation
- diarrhea
- gas
- heartburn
- nausea
- vomiting
- dizziness

(Continued)

(Continued)

Get emergency help right away if you have any of the following symptoms:

- shortness of breath or trouble breathing
- chest pain
- weakness in one part or side of your body
- slurred speech
- swelling of the face or throat

Stop your NSAID medicine and call your healthcare provider right away if you have any of the following symptoms:

- nausea
- more tired or weaker than usual
- itching
- your skin or eyes look yellow
- stomach pain
- flu-like symptoms
- vomit blood
- there is blood in your bowel movement or it is black and sticky like tar
- skin rash or blisters with fever
- unusual weight gain
- swelling of the arms and legs, hands and feet

These are not all the side effects with NSAID medicines. Talk to your healthcare provider or pharmacist for more information about NSAID medicines.

Other information about Non-Steroidal Anti-Inflammatory Drugs (NSAIDs)
Aspirin is an NSAID medicine but it does not increase the chance of a heart attack. Aspirin can cause bleeding in the brain, stomach, and intestines. Aspirin can also cause ulcers in the stomach and intestines. Some of these NSAID medicines are sold in lower doses without a prescription (over-the-counter). Talk to your healthcare provider before using over-the-counter NSAIDs for more than 10 days.

NSAID medicines that need a prescription

Generic Name	Tradename
Celecoxib	Celebrex
Diclofenac	Cataflam, Voltaren, Arthrotec (combined with misoprostol)
Diflunisal	Dolobid
Etodolac	Lodine, Lodine XL
Fenoprofen	Nalfon, Nalfon 200
Flurbiprofen	Ansaid
Ibuprofen	Motrin, Tab-Profen, Vicoprofen* (combined with hydrocodone), Combunox (combined with oxycodone)
Indomethacin	Indocin, Indocin SR, Indo-Lemmon, Indomethagan
Ketoprofen	Oruvail
Ketorolac	Toradol
Mefenamic Acid	Ponstel
Meloxicam	Mobic
Nabumetone	Relafen
Naproxen	Naprosyn, Anaprox, Anaprox DS, EC-Naprosyn, Naprelan, PREVACID NapraPAC (copackaged with lansoprazole)
Oxaprozin	Daypro
Piroxicam	Feldene
Sulindac	Clinoril
Tolmetin	Tolectin, Tolectin DS, Tolectin 600

*Vicoprofen contains the same dose of ibuprofen as over-the-counter (OTC) NSAIDs, and is usually used for less than 10 days to treat pain. The OTC NSAID label warns that long term continuous use may increase the risk of heart attack or stroke.

This Medication Guide has been approved by the U.S. Food and Drug Administration.

GI Risks With NSAIDs

One of the major risks with nonselective NSAIDs is gastric ulceration. Gastric ulcers develop within a week in about 30% of patients started on nonselective NSAIDs (Wallace & Staats, 2005). Most patients with these ulcers are asymptomatic and only seek medical care when the bleeding becomes obvious with tarry stools or hematemesis.

Some practitioners prescribe proton pump inhibitors (PPI), such as omeprazole (Prilosec), which only provides protection for the upper GI system. Patient compliance with PPI for protection is also suspect. A recent study found that by the time the patients received three prescriptions for a PPI as NSAID prophylaxis, the nonadherence rate for patients with PPIs was high at 60.8% (D'Arcy, 2010; Sturkenboom, 2003).

Some older patients are also using an aspirin a day for cardioprotective effect, adding the incidence of ulcer formation with aspirin to the NSAID risk only increases the potential for GI bleeding. Patients who use higher doses and are older have an increased occurrence rate of GI side effects (Perez-Gutthann, 1997). Higher doses and older age are associated with a higher incidence of GI side effects (Perez-Gutthann, 1997). Additionally, chronic alcohol use with NSAIDs increases the risk of GI bleeding and ulceration. Deciding if NSAIDs are an appropriate treatment option for the patient depends largely on the individual patient's history and medical situation.

Cardiovascular Risks With NSAIDs

For patients who have had recent heart bypass surgery, patients with heart disease, and patients who have had transient ischemic attacks or strokes, NSAID use presents a higher risk for cardiovascular events and their use is not recommended (Bennett et al., 2005). For these patients, an alternate form of analgesic is recommended.

When trying to determine if NSAIDs are a good treatment option, consider that naproxen interferes with the inhibitory effect of aspirin (Capone, Sciulli, & Tacconelli, 2005) and that similar effects may be seen with concomitant use of ibuprofen (Advil, Motrin), acetaminophen (Tylenol), and diclofenac (Cataflam, Voltaren) (Catella-Lawson, Reilly, & Kapoor, 2001). Weighing the risk and benefits of using NSAIDs for a patient who is using aspirin for cardiac prophylaxis should include the consideration of an increased risk of GI events and the aspirin effectiveness may be decreased.

Overall, the recommendations for using NSAIDs for pain relief indicate that the medication should be used at the lowest dose for the shortest time (Bennett et al., 2005). For older patients this means that long-term use of NSAIDs for chronic conditions such as arthritis can lead to serious and even life-threatening events.

New Developments With NSAIDs

Newer forms of NSAIDs have come to market recently. These types of NSAIDs are called targeted topical medications and are applied directly at the site of pain. Some of the medications are applied as liquids, whereas others have been made into patches. The newest formulation is a liquid made of diclofenac sodium, a topical solution called Pennsaid. The liquid can be applied directly to the knees for patients with osteoarthritis. Diclofenac also comes as a 1% gel formulation that is rapidly absorbed and is recommended for use on joints with osteoarthritis. The patient will need to apply the solution or gel to the affected joint four times per day for maximum pain relief.

A patch containing 1% of diclofenac epolamine (Flector) has been used successfully for minor orthopedic injuries, such as strains and sprains. The patch should be applied directly to the site of the injury. Despite the topical application, each medication has recommendations to use the smallest dose possible for the shortest time, and gastrointestinal effect, though rare, cannot be excluded.

Case Study

Cecelia P. is a 65-year-old retired school teacher who has osteoarthritis in her knees and has recently been complaining about new back pain. Her back pain started 2 weeks ago after she worked in her garden pulling weeds. She tried to treat the pain at home with acetaminophen and some Advil, but she is still having difficulty moving around her house. The pain is constant and achy, and she rates it at 6/10. She comes into your office asking for help with her pain. How will you help Cecelia with her pain?

Questions to Consider

1. Is her back pain inflammatory or musculoskeletal?
2. Cecelia's knee pain is inflammatory. What medications could you recommend for her if she has a history of gastroesophageal reflux disease (GERD) and hypertension?
3. Would you consider any of the new targeted medications, such as a Flector patch, for the back pain?
4. Would acetaminophen or aspirin be good choices for the back pain the patient is experiencing?
5. How will you educate Cecelia about taking over-the-counter medications considering her GERD and hypertension?

REFERENCES

Alazraki, M. (2009). *Raw risk of over-the-counter meds: How many Tylenols have you taken today?* Retrieved from http://www.dailyfinance.com/

American Geriatrics Society (AGS). (2002). Panel on persistent pain in older persons. *Journal of the American Geriatrics Society, 50*(6), 1–20.

American Geriatrics Society (AGS). (2009). Pharmacological management of persistent pain in older persons. *Journal of the American Geriatrics Society, 57*(8), 1331–1346.

Bennett, J. S., Daugherty, A., Herrington, D., Greenland, P., Roberts, H., & Taubert, K. A. (2005). The use of nonsteroidal anti-inflammatory drugs (NSAIDs): A science advisory from the American Heart Association. *Circulation, 111*(13), 1713–1716.

Brennan, F., Carr, D. B., & Cousins, M. (2007). Pain management: A fundamental human right. *Anesthesia & Analgesia, 105*(1), 205–221.

Bruckenthal, P. (2007). Controlled substances: Principles of safe prescribing. *The Nurse Practitioner, 32*(5), 7–11.

Buvanendran, A., & Lipman, A. (2009). Nonsteroidal anti-inflammatory drugs and acetaminophen. In J. Ballantyne, S. Fishman, & J. Rathmell (Eds.), *Bonica's management of pain* (4th ed., pp. 1157–1171). Philadelphia: Lippincott Williams and Wilkins.

Capone, M. L., Sciulli, M. G., Tacconelli, S., Grana, M., Ricciotti, M., Renda, G., . . . Patrignani, P. (2005). Pharmacodynamic interaction of naproxen with low-dose aspirin in healthy subjects. *Journal of the College of Cardiology, 45*(8), 1295–1301.

Catella-Lawson, F., Reilly, M., Kapoor, S., Cucchiara, A., DeMarco, S., Tournier, B., . . . FitzGerald, G. (2001). Cyclooxygenase inhibitors and the antiplatelet effects of aspirin. *New England Journal of Medicine, 345*(25), 1809–1817.

Chou, R., Fanciullo, G. J., Fine, P. G., Adler, J. A., Ballantyne, J. C., Davies, P., . . . Miaskowski, C. (2009). Clinical guidelines for the use of chronic opioid therapy in chronic noncancer pain. *The Journal of Pain, 10*(2), 113–130.

D'Arcy, Y. (2007). *Pain management: Evidence based tools and techniques for nursing professionals*. Marblehead, MA: HCPro.

D'Arcy, Y. (2009a). Be in the know about pain management. *The Nurse Practitioner, 34*(4), 43–47.

D'Arcy, Y. (2009b). Opioid therapy: Focus on patient safety. *American Nurse Today, 495*, 18–22.

D'Arcy, Y. (2009c). Treating low back pain with evidence-based options. *The Nurse Practitioner.*

Institute for Clinical Systems Improvement. (2008). *Assessment and management of chronic pain*. Bloomington, MN: Author.

Karani, R., & Meier, D. (2004). Systematic pharmacologic postoperative pain management in the geriatric orthopaedic patient. *Clinical Orthopaedics and Related Research, 425*, 26–34.

Miaskowski C., Bair, M., Chou, R., D'Arcy, Y., Hartwick, C., Huffman, L., . . . Manwarren, R. (2008). *Principles of analgesic use in the treatment of acute pain and cancer pain* (6th ed.). Glenview, IL: American Pain Society.

Nursing 2010 Drug Handbook. (2009). Philadelphia: Wolters Kluwer/ Lippincott Williams and Wilkins.

Pan, G. J. D. (2009). *Acetaminophen: Background and overview.* Retrieved from www.fda.gov.

Perez-Gutthann, S., Garcia Rodriguez, L., & Raiford, D. S. (1997) Individual nonsteroidal anti-inflammatory drugs and other risk factors for upper gastrointestinal bleeding and perforation. *Epidemiology, 8*, 18–24.

Stanos, S. P., Fishbain, D. A., & Fishman, S. M. (2009). Pain management with opioid analgesics: Balancing risk and benefit. *Physical Medicine & Rehabilitation, 88*(3, Suppl. 2), S69–S99.

Sturkenboom, M. C., Burke, T. A., Tangelder, M. J., Dieleman, J. P., Walton, S., & Goldstein, J. L. (2003). Adherence to proton pump inhibitors or H2-receptor antagonists during the use of non-steroidal anti-inflammatory drugs. *Alimentary Pharmacology and Therapeutics, 18*(11–12), 1137–1147.

Trescot, A. M., Helm, S., Hansen, H., Benyamin, R., Glaser, S. E., Adlaka, R., . . . Manchikanti, L. (2008). Opioids in the management of chronic non-cancer pain: An update of American Society of Interventional Pain Physicians' (ASIPP) guidelines. *Pain Physician, 11*(Suppl. 2), S5–S62.

Wallace, M., & Staats, P. (2005). *Pain medicine and management.* New York, NY: McGraw-Hill.

ADDITIONAL RESOURCES

Chu, L. F., Clark, D. J., & Angst, M. S. (2006). Opioid tolerance and hyperalgesia in chronic pain patients after one month of oral morphine therapy: A preliminary prospective study. *The Journal of Pain, 7*(1), 43–48.

Dworkin, R. H., O'Connor, A. B., Backonja, M., Farrar, J. T., Finnerup, N. B., Jensen, T. S., . . . Wallace, M. S. (2007). Pharmacologic management of neuropathic pain: Evidence-based recommendations. *Pain, 132*(3), 237–251.

Fine, P., & Portnoy, R. (2007). *A clinical guide to opioid analgesia.* New York: Vendome Group Health Care.

Veterans Health Administration, Department of Defense. (2003). *VA/DoD clinical practice guideline for the management of opioids therapy for chronic pain.* Washington, DC: Author.

7

Opioid Analgesics

OVERVIEW OF OPIOID MEDICATIONS

Opioids are medications that are derived from the opium poppy, *Papaver somniferum*. They have a long history of pain relief and have been used in various forms, such as elixirs and potions, and also smoked since the time of the Sumerians; in that culture, the poppy was depicted in art as "the plant of joy" (Osler, cited in Fine & Portnoy, 2007). Reports from early Greek, Egyptian, and Roman societies described the fact that many of the leaders and everyday citizens used opium for pain relief. In the 16th century, the use of laudanum, an opium-derived elixir, was common for various pain complaints. It was during this time that dependence and tolerance were first observed to be occurring in laudanum users. In the early days of the United States, cocaine-containing elixirs and tonics for pain relief were sold by peddlers. Laudanum was a major pain reliever for households in the Civil War era of the 1860s.

The term *opioid* or *opiate* denotes a class of medications that are derived from the latex sap of the opium poppy or created as analogs to these natural substances. Opium has a two-sided history: one as a potent analgesic and the other as a recreational drug. For example, it was smoked for its euphoric effect in the opium dens of China and also used for pain relief. Early herbalists recognized the analgesic potential of opium and used it to treat many different types of pain in their patients.

During the 19th century, China's trade with the British consisted of large amounts of opium. The supply was high and demand for the product was just as great, leading to wars and infighting over the use of opium to balance trade. Morphine was first isolated in 1895 in Germany, where the medication was thought to be useful as a cure for opium addiction (McCoy, cited in Fine & Portnoy, 2007). The development of the hypodermic syringe in the mid-19th century gave medical practitioners another route for delivering opioid medications that they injected directly into the site of the pain.

By the 20th century, opioid use not only was seen as beneficial for treating pain but also had become problematic as opioid abuse increased. The United States passed the first two acts for controlling the use of opioids: the Pure Food and Drug Act (1906) and the Harrison Narcotics Act (1914). As late as 1970, the Federal Controlled Substances Act provided standards for the monitoring, manufacturing, prescribing, and dispensing of opioids and created the five-level division of controlled substances that we use today.

In general, opioids are some of the best medications we have to control pain. They come in various formulations and have few adverse side effects when compared with other medication types.

Natural derivatives of opium include morphine, codeine, and heroin. Synthetic analogues, such as fentanyl (Sublimaze) and meperidine (Demerol), were developed much later as attempts to perfect compounds for better pain relief. All of the opioid compounds share certain features.

- They activate by binding sites in the body called mu receptors to produce analgesia. Mu receptors are found in many places in the body, including the brain and spinal column neurons.
- Their main action is analgesia.
- Side effects, such as sedation, constipation, and nausea, are common.
- They all are potentially addicting. Analgesia is the goal of opioid administration. The cytocrome P450 system, located in the liver, transforms some opioids into usable metabolites (Fine & Portnoy, 2007). The rate that opioids are metabolized varies from person to person, with the range being ultraslow to ultrarapid. Additionally, 5% to 10% of Caucasians lack the ability or have poor ability to

convert codeine to morphine (Løvlie et al., 2001). In some older individuals, changes in proteins may limit the binding ability of opioid medications (Zurakowski, 2009).

The Various Forms of Opioids

Some opioids are used in the natural form, such as morphine and heroin. Other natural opium alkaloids include codeine, noscapine, papaverine, and thebaine. These alkaloids can be further reduced into more common analgesic compounds. The alkaloid thebaine is used to produce semisynthetic opioid morphine analogues, such as oxycodone (Percocet, Percodan), hydromorphone (Dilaudid), hydrocodone (Vicodin/Lortab), and etorphine (Immobilon). Other classes of morphine analogues include the 4-diphenylpiperidines: meperidine (Demerol), diphenylpropylamines, and methadone (Dolophine). Each of these compounds was developed to either increase analgesic effect or reduce the potential for addiction.

Although all of the opioid substances can be classed as pain relievers, their potency varies. Etorphine is one of the most potent of the analogue compounds, with very small amounts providing a great effect. Each member of the morphine group has one chemical similarity. There must be a piperidine ring in the chemical configuration or a greater part of the ring must be chemically present to be classified as a morphine.

The main binding sites for opioids, the mu receptors (Holden, Jeong, & Forrest, 2005), are found in the following areas:

- Brain cortex
- Thalamus
- Periaqueductal gray matter
- Spinal cord substantia gelatinosa (Fine & Portnoy, 2007)

Other secondary binding sites include the kappa and delta sites. Kappa sites are found in the brain's hypothalamus, periaqueductal gray matter, claustrum, and spinal cord substantia gelatinosa. The delta receptors are located in the pontine nucleus, amygdala, olfactory bulbs, and the deep cortex of the brain. Recently, an opioid

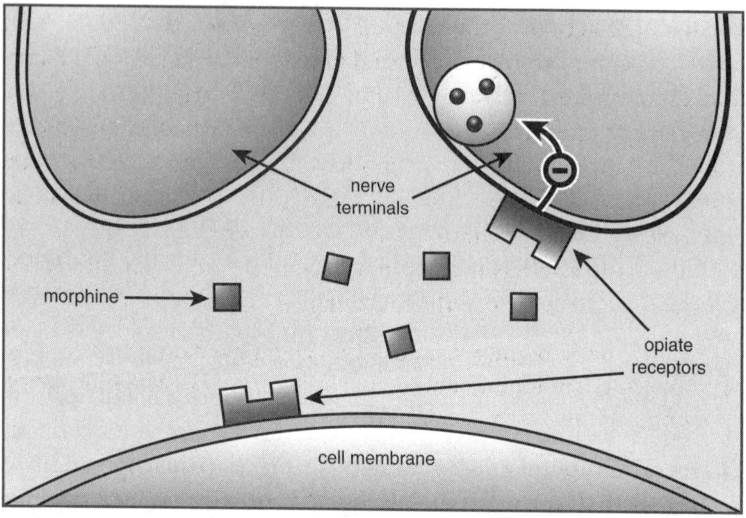

Figure 7.1 ■ Opioid receptor-like 1 site

receptor-like site was discovered and named opioid receptor-like 1 (Figure 7.1). The activity at this site is thought to be related to central modulation of pain but does not appear to have an effect on respiratory depression (Fine & Portnoy, 2007).

When an opioid is introduced into a patient's body, it looks for the binding site that conforms to a specific protein pattern that will allow the opioid to bind to the receptor site and create analgesia, an agonist action. At one time, the binding action for opioids was believed to be a simple lock-and-key effect: introduce the medication, find the binding site, and bind, thus creating analgesia. Today, we know that the process is much more specific and is more sophisticated than a simple lock-and-key model.

Once the opioid molecule approaches the cell, it looks for a way to bind. On the exterior of each cell are ligands, or cellular channel mechanisms, connecting the exterior of the cell with the interior and conveying the opioid molecule into the cell. The ligands are affiliated with the exterior receptor sites and can contain various G-proteins. These G-proteins couple with the opioid molecule and mediate the action of the receptor (Fine & Portnoy, 2007). "One opioid receptor can regulate several G proteins, and multiple receptors can activate a single G protein" (Fine & Portnoy, 2007, p. 11). As efforts progress to better identify the process, more than 40 variations in binding site composition have been identified (Pasternak, 2005). These differences explain some of the variation in patient response to opioid medications.

The body also has natural pain-facilitating and pain-inhibiting substances. These include the following:

- Facilitating: substance P, bradykinin, and glutamate
- Inhibiting: serotonin, natural or synthetic opioids, norepinephrine, gamma-aminobutyric acid (GABA)

When these substances are activated or blocked, pain can be relieved or increased. These more complex mechanisms are difficult to tease out, and trying to link them to analgesia and opioid effect can be misguided. More information on pain-facilitating and pain-inhibiting substances can be found in Chapter 1.

Types of Opioid Medications

Opioid medications are very versatile in that they can be given as a standalone medication, such as codeine, or combined with another type of nonopioid medication, such as a nonsteroidal anti-inflammatory drug (NSAID; e.g., ibuprofen [Combunox] or acetaminophen [Tylenol #3 or Percocet]). Some of the medications have elixirs, such as morphine (Roxanol), and others have a suppository form, such as hydromorphone (Dilaudid). Because the elixir form can be very bitter, adding a flavoring available at most pharmacies can help the patient tolerate the taste of the medication.

The duration of the oral short-acting preparations is usually listed as 4 to 6 hours, but each patient has an individual response and ability to metabolize medications. Most of the combination medications are considered short acting, and the combination of another type of medication such as acetaminophen limits the amount of medication that can be taken in a 24-hour period. Preparations in which opioids are combined with acetaminophen follow the recommended dose for daily acetaminophen use to 4,000 mg/day maximum (American Pain Society [APS], 2008).

Other medications, especially those on the third level of the World Health Organization analgesic ladder, have extended-release (ER) formulations. These ER formulations not only make the medication a pure opioid agonist alone but also, when ER formulations are used, the dosing time is extended to 12 to 24 hours, such as with ER morphines (MS Contin, Avinza, Kadian) or ER oxycodone (Oxycontin). These ER medications are particularly helpful for patients in whom pain is present throughout the day, such as patients with chronic pain and patients with cancer. These ER medications are not designed to be used in patients with acute pain who are opioid naïve (patients who have not been taking opioid medications), but for those who have been taking the short-acting medications regularly to control their pain.

Some long-acting opioid medications, such as the fentanyl patch (Duragesic), have specific short-acting medication requirements before they can be used (e.g., before using Duragesic 25 mg, the patient must have been using the opioid equivalent of Dilaudid 8 mg by mouth per day for 2 weeks prior to patch application). Every patient who uses an ER opioid medication for pain should have a short-acting medication to use for breakthrough pain that occurs with increased activity or for end-of-dose failure that allows pain levels to increase (APS, 2008).

No matter what type or form of opioid medication is being considered for use, the health care provider should be aware of the risks and benefits of each medication and weigh the options carefully. A full history and physical and risk assessment for opioid therapy should be performed.

Short-Acting Combination Medications

Short-acting pain medications come in a wide variety of types. Some are combined with acetaminophen or other nonopioid medications and others are opioid medications, such as oxycodone, that only last for several hours at the recommended doses. For most patients with an acute injury, such as surgery, a short-acting medication is appropriate, and the patient will use it intermittently throughout the period of recovery. Once the surgical pain resolves, the patient no longer needs to take the opioid medication and should stop medication use. Patients with chronic pain require a more complex medication regimen to control their pain effectively, especially if the chronic pain is an underlying condition to an acute pain presentation.

Most short-acting medications are oral, as either pills or elixirs. For surgical pain, a short-acting medication may be needed in the immediate postoperative period, and these are given as intermittent intravenous (IV) doses or through patient-controlled analgesia (PCA). One route of administration that is no longer recommended is the intramuscular (IM) injection. Because the administration of medication via the IM route allows for irregular absorption of the medication and tissue sclerosis, most national guidelines and pain specialists have eliminated the IM route from their recommendations (APS, 2008; ASPMN, 2010).

Conversely, for patients with chronic pain, the pain will continue with no end point and so medication use will continue. For these patients, a careful assessment of pain patterns and intensities throughout the day will help determine when and how the opioid medication will be prescribed. If the pain is only episodic or present at certain times of day, a short-acting medication may provide all the pain relief that is needed. However, most patients with chronic pain have pain that is continuous, so adding an ER medication is common.

Most short-acting opioid medications are designed for moderate to severe pain intensities. Onset of action is usually 10 to 60 minutes with a short duration of action of 2 to 4 hours (Katz, McCarberg, & Reisner, 2007). Overall advantages to short-acting medications include a synergistic effect with the combination of medications that can improve pain relief and provide a better outcome.

MEDICATIONS

Short-Acting Combination Medications: Intermittent Pain, Breakthrough Pain

■ *Codeine-Containing Medications: Codeine, Tylenol #3 (Codeine 30 mg Combined With Acetaminophen 325 mg)*

Used to treat mild to moderate pain, codeine[1] is noted to have a "number needed to treat" of 11. That means the first effective analgesic effect would be seen in the 12th patient who was given the medication for pain relief. About 10% of the people lack the enzyme needed to activate codeine (APS, 2008). Codeine has a high profile for side effects, such as constipation, and gastrointestinal (GI) disturbances, such as nausea and vomiting (APS, 2008). It is often used as a component in cough syrups as a cough suppressant (*Nursing 2010 Drug Handbook*, 2009). The medication can also be given in an elixir form, which is convenient for patients who have difficulty swallowing or for use with enteral feeding tubes.

■ *Hydrocodone-Containing Medications: Vicodin, Lortab, Norco, and Lortab Elixir*

Hydrocodone-containing medications are designed to be used for moderate pain. They usually contain 5 to 10 mg of hydrocodone with 325 mg or 500 mg of acetaminophen. Many patients tolerate the medication very well for intermittent pain or for breakthrough pain. It is available in an elixir form that is very effective and can be used with patients who have difficulty swallowing pills or for use with enteral feeding tubes. Norco has a higher dose of hydrocodone per tablet.

■ *Oxycodone-Containing Medications: Oxycodone, Percocet, Roxicet, Percodan, and Oxfast*

Medications with oxycodone are designed for treating moderate-level pain. They are commonly used for postoperative pain in the acute care setting and for patients with chronic pain. Percocet is a combination medication with 5 mg of oxycodone and 325 mg of acetaminophen. Percodan

---

[1] Codeine should be used with caution in breastfeeding women who may inadvertently give their infants a morphine overdose if they are ultrarapid codeine metabolizers (*Nursing 2010 Drug Handbook*, 2009).

is a combination of oxycodone and aspirin. If the patient requires a higher dose of medication for pain control, combining an oxycodone 5 mg tablet with a combined form such as Roxicet will provide additional pain relief but still maintain the acetaminophen dose at 325 mg. To help patients tolerate the medication without nausea, giving the medication with milk or after meals is recommended (*Nursing 2010 Drug Handbook*, 2009).

Oxymorphone-Containing Medications: Opana

Opana is a medication designed to treat moderate to severe pain. It has a more extended half-life than other medications of the same class, resulting in a decreased need for breakthrough medications (Adams et al., 2004; Adams & Abdieh, 2005). Opana should be taken 1 hour before or 2 hours after a meal (*Nursing 2010 Drug Handbook*, 2009). It is also available in an injectable form for use during labor (*Nursing 2010 Drug Handbook*, 2009).

Tramadol: Ultram and Ultracet

Tramadol is a unique medication that combines a mu agonist, an opioid-like medication, and selective serotonin reuptake inhibitor-type medication. It is designed for use with moderate pain. Doses should be reduced for older patients and in patients with increased creatinine levels or cirrhosis. Tramadol may increase the risk of seizures and serotonin syndrome (*Nursing 2010 Drug Handbook*, 2009). Patients should be instructed to taper off the medication gradually when discontinuing it. It should not be stopped suddenly (*Nursing 2010 Drug Handbook*, 2009). Tapentadol (Nucynta) is a medication similar to tramadol. It has a dual action of mu agonism but it also has a selective serotonin and norepinephrine reuptake inhibitor action with a lessened serotonin effect when compared to tramadol. It is indicated for acute pain and may have some activity for neuropathic pain. Dose adjustment should be made for elderly and patients with renal or hepatic dysfunction.

Hydromorphone: Dilaudid

Dilaudid is an extremely potent analgesic and it is designed for use with severe level pain. In the oral form, it comes in 2 mg and 4 mg tablets. In the IV form, 0.2 mg of Dilaudid is equal to 1 mg of intravenous morphine. Dilaudid is a medication that is commonly used only after the other medications for pain (e.g., Vicodin and Percocet) are trialed unsuccessfully.

Because of the strength of this medication, it is possible to get good pain relief with small amounts and to potentially have fewer side effects. See Chapter 12 for PCA use.

■ *Morphine: Immediate-Release Morphine (MSIR) and Roxanol (Elixir)*

Morphine is the gold standard for severe level pain relief. It is the standard for equianalgesic conversions and has a long history of use for pain control. It is available in many different forms: pills, elixir, IV, and suppository. The biggest drawback to morphine is the side effect profile; constipation, nausea and vomiting, delirium, and hallucinations are some of the most commonly reported adverse effects.

■ *Fentanyl Transmucosal (Sublimaze): Actiq, Fentora, and Onsolis*

There is no oral pill formulation possible for fentanyl. The route of administration is either transdermal or buccal. When used buccally for breakthrough or incident pain in opioid-tolerant patients (patients who take opioid medications regularly), the transmucosal medications can be rubbed across the buccal membrane and absorbed directly into the cardiac circulation. Fentanyl's fast absorption rate makes this medication a risk for oversedation, so the indication is only for breakthrough pain in opioid-tolerant cancer patients or patients with chronic pain who take opioid medications on a daily basis.

If the entire dose of an Actiq oralet is not used, it should be placed in a childproof container until the remainder is needed. This medication as patch or oral form is not intended to be used for acute or postoperative pain (*Nursing 2010 Drug Handbook*, 2009). It is not meant to be used in opioid-naïve patients because serious oversedation can occur (Fine & Portnoy, 2007). If a patient with chronic pain or cancer pain is having surgery or has another acute pain complaint and he or she is using buccal fentanyl for pain control, care must be taken in providing IV pain medications to avoid oversedation.

Extended-Release (ER) Medications: Around-the-Clock Pain Relief

For opioid-tolerant patients or patients with chronic pain, ER medication can give a consistent blood level of medication, providing a steady comfort level. This may increase functionality and improve quality of life, enhance sleep, and let the patient participate in meaningful daily activities. ER medications have a slower onset of action from 30 to 90 minutes with a relatively long duration of action of up to 72 hours (Katz, McCarberg, & Reisner, 2007).

When a patient has pain that lasts throughout the day and the patient is taking short-acting medications and has reached the maximum dose limitations of the nonopioid medication, the prescriber should consider switching the patient to an ER or long-acting medication. Candidates for this type of therapy in acute care are trauma patients with extensive orthopedic injuries who will require long-term rehabilitation and will need to have tolerable pain to participate in their recovery.

Some of the short-acting medications have an ER formulation, including Vicodin ER, Opana ER, Ultram ER, Oxycontin, Exalgo, Kadian, Avinza, and MS Contin. Most are pure mu agonist medications, such as morphine, with an ER action that allows the medication to dissolve slowly in the GI tract. Some ER medications are encapsulated into beads that allow gastric secretions to enter the bead and force the medication out. Other ER formulations have a coating around an ER plasticized compound that keeps the medication from dissolving too quickly. Most ER medications either have or are developing a formula that makes them more tamper resistant to avoid improper use. When ER medication is being started with a patient, the patient should be instructed on the important aspects of the medications. Important information includes the following:

- ER medications of all types should never be broken, chewed, or degraded in any way to enhance the absorption of the medications. To do so risks all the medication being given at one time, and there is then a high risk of potentially fatal oversedation.
- Most ER medications should not be taken with alcohol. To do so degrades the ER mechanism and allows for a faster absorption of the medication, which can cause potentially fatal oversedation.
- ER medications are not meant to be injected.
- ER medications should not be crushed and inserted into enteral feeding tubes.

- ER medications are not meant to be used on an as-needed basis, but rather as scheduled daily doses.
- If the patient experiences end-of-dose failure several hours before the next dose of medication is due, the interval should be shortened or more common the dose should be increased (APS, 2008).

When converting a patient from short-acting medications, the rule of thumb are as follows:

- If the medication is the same (e.g., Percocet to Oxycontin), equivalent doses of the medication can be prescribed.
- If the medication is a different drug (e.g., Percocet to MS Contin), the daily dose should be calculated using the equianalgesic conversion table (see Table 7.1) and reduced usually by 30%. To ensure adequate pain relief is maintained, additional doses of breakthrough medication should be prescribed about 5% to 15% of the total daily dose to be taken every 2 hours as needed (APS, 2008).

Methadone: Dolophine and Methadose

Methadone is considered to be a long-acting medication because it has an extended half-life of 15 to 60 hours (APS, 2008). Pain relief for the oral form, however, is less extended at 4 to 6 hours (*Nursing 2010 Drug Handbook*, 2009). Therein lies the danger. Given that the half-life is very long and the pain relief is shorter, dosing must be done very carefully to avoid oversedation, which may become apparent only a day or two after the doses are given. Dose escalation should be done no more often than every 3 to 7 days (APS, 2008).

Methadone can be prescribed legally by general practitioners in primary care and acute care for pain relief. It is also used for methadone maintenance to control addiction in heroin addicts. To prescribe methadone for these patients requires a special licensure. The addiction program has no connection to prescribing methadone for pain management. However, because there is such a risk with methadone, the current recommendation of the APS is that only pain management practitioners or those skilled and knowledgeable about the medication prescribe the drug (APS, 2008).

An additional risk factor for methadone is the potential for QT corrected interval prolongation and, at higher doses, for torsades de pointes (APS, 2008). Primary care providers are advised to obtain a baseline electrocardiogram (ECG) for patients who are on daily methadone

Table 7.1 ■ *Equianalgesic Table for Opioid Conversion*

Analgesics	*Generic*	*Brand Name*	*Oral dose*	*Parenteral*	
Immediate release	Morphine	Roxanol, MSIR	30 milligrams	10 milligrams	Relative potency 1:6 with acute dosing and 1:2 to 1:3 with chronic dosing
	Oxycodone	Roxicodone, Oxy IR	20 milligrams	NA	
	Hydromorphone	Dilaudid	7.5 milligrams	1.5 milligrams	
	Oxymorphone	Opana, Numorphan	10 milligrams	1 milligram	Extended half life with short-acting oral form
	Hydrocodone	Vicodin, Lortab	30 milligrams	NA	
	Fentanyl	Sublimaze	NA	100 micrograms	
	Methadone	Dolophine	5-10 milligrams	10 milligrams	Use with caution: Half life of 12-150 hours accumulates with repeated dosing
	Meperidine	Demerol	NR	NR	Use with caution. Toxic metabolite normeperidine can cause seizures
Controlled Release	*Generic*	*Brand Name*	*Oral dose*	*Parenteral*	
Not recommended for opioid-naïve patients	Morphine	MSContin, Avinza, Kadian	20-30		
	Oxycodone	Oxycontin	20-30 milligrams		
	Fentanyl transdermal	Duragesic	NA	25 micrograms	

Basic Intravenous conversion: Morphine 1 milligram = Dilaudid 0.2 milligrams = Fentanyl 10 micrograms
NR = not recommended
When switching from one opioid to another, reduce the dose by 25% to 50% with adequate breakthrough medication
When switching to methadone, reduce the equianalgesic dose by 75% to 90%
Breakthrough medication should be available when controlled release medications are being used
All opioid medications should be carefully dosed and titrated with consideration for the individual patient and the medical condition of the patient
Sources: American Pain Society. (2008). *Principles of Analgesic Use in the Treatment of Acute Pain and Cancer Pain;* Fine, P., & Portnoy, R. (2007). *Opioid Analgesia;* Inturrisi, C., & Lipman, A. (2010). *Bonica's Management of Pain,* pp. 1174–1175; Smith, H., & McCleane, G. (2009). *Current Therapy in Pain.*
Used with permission of the author.

and continue to obtain regular ECGs as the doses escalate more than 200 mg/day (APS, 2008).

■ *Fentanyl Patches: Duragesic*

Fentanyl patches can provide a high level of pain relief and are used for various chronic pain conditions. Patches are the only transdermal opioid application available for use. The Duragesic patch is a delivery system that contains a specified dose of fentanyl in a gel formulation. It is designed for use with opioid-tolerant patients and should never be used for acute pain or with opioid-naïve patients.

The patch is applied to clean intact skin and delivers the specified amount of medication over a period of 72 hours (e.g., 25 mcg/hr). The medication effect begins as the medication depot develops in the subcutaneous fat, and it can take from 12 to 18 hours for pain relief to begin (D'Arcy, 2007, 2009a). It can also take up to 48 hours for steady-state blood levels to develop so when the patch is being started, the patient will need additional breakthrough pain medication (D'Arcy, 2009a).

There are some safety concerns with Duragesic patch use. More than 100 patients have died related to fentanyl patch use and misuse. When a patch is prescribed for pain relief, patient education should include the following points:

- Do not cut the patch. To do so will result in a dose-dumping effect where all the medication is released at one time, resulting in an overdose.
- Do not apply heat over the patch. To do so may result in accelerated medication delivery, also resulting in potential overdose.
- Dispose of the patch in a closed container, flush it down a toilet, or seal it in a sealable bag with kitty litter or used coffee grounds. Because there is medication left in the patch, safe disposal is necessary to avoid diversion and minimize contamination.
- Do not place the patch in a regular wastebasket when discarding it. There is about 16% of the dose remaining in the patch after use and a small animal or child could remove the patch and chew or come in contact with it.

Before a 25 mcg fentanyl patch is placed, the patient should be taking one of the following: 30 mg of oxycodone per day for 2 weeks, 8 mg of hydromorphone per day for 2 weeks, or 60 mg of oral morphine per day for 2 weeks (Janssen prescribing information available at www.Janssen.com).

Medications That Are No Longer Recommended

There are two pain medications that are no longer recommended for use related to toxic metabolites, high acetaminophen doses, or high profile for side effects.

■ *Propoxyphene With Acetaminophen: Darvocet*

Darvocet is a medication that has fallen out of favor and is being considered for withdrawal by the U.S. Food and Drug Administration because of the high levels of acetaminophen. It is designed to treat mild level pain, but its analgesic action is created primarily by the high dose of acetaminophen it contains. Each tablet contains 650 mg of acetaminophen and 50 or 100 mg of propoxyphene. It is very easy to reach daily maximum doses of acetaminophen with just a few tablets of Darvocet. Additionally, there is a toxic metabolite called norpropoxyphene that can build up with use and can cause seizures (APS, 2008). For these reasons, it is not used very often by pain specialists for pain control, and it is not recommended for patients with renal impairment or in older adults (APS, 2008). As of December 2010 this medication has been removed from the market by the FDA.

■ *Meperidine: Demerol*

Meperidine (Demerol) has also fallen out of favor. It is no longer considered a first-line pain medication (APS, 2008; D'Arcy, 2007). Meperidine has a toxic metabolite called normeperidine that accumulates with repetitive dosing (APS,2008). This metabolite can cause tremors and seizures. Other drawbacks include the need to use high doses to achieve an analgesic effect that is accompanied by sedation and nausea (D'Arcy, 2007). If Demerol is going to be used, there are certain recommendations that include the following:

- Demerol should never be used in children and infants.
- It should never be used in patients with renal impairment (e.g., older patients or patients with sickle cell disease).
- Hyperpyrexic syndrome with delirium can occur if Demerol is used in patients who are taking monoamine oxidase inhibitors, which can be potentially fatal.
- If used, it should never be administered for more than 1 to 2 days at doses not to exceed 600 mg/24 hr (APS, 2008).

Mixed Agonists/Antagonist Medications

There is a group of medications that have both an agonist and an antagonist action at the various binding sites throughout the body. These medications are called *mixed agonist/antagonist medications* and include the following:

- Nubain
- Talwin
- Buprenex

These medications act further down on the spinal cord at the kappa receptor sites, so there is less potential for respiratory depression. Because these medications have both agonist and antagonist action, they have the potential for reversing the opioid effect of pure opioid agonists, such as morphine. If a patient is taking morphine, giving a mixed agonist/antagonist medication will reverse the analgesic effect of the morphine and pain relief is lessened. This group of medications also has a high profile for adverse side effects, such as confusion and hallucinations, and has dose ceilings that limit dose escalations (APS, 2008).

Selecting an Opioid

Selecting an opioid for an individual patient can involve a trial-and-error process. Each individual has a genetic preference for one or more types of opioids. Which opioid works best for the patient must be determined. For most patients who are hospitalized and have severe pain, the analgesic will need to be administered by the IV route. For other patients with acute injuries, a short-acting oral medication may be enough to control the pain (Table 7.2).

Many patients with pain have tried opioids before. They may know which opioid works best and which ones do not work at all. If the patient can provide you with information on the efficacy of pain medications, it should not be considered as drug seeking or potential addiction. If a patient has used a medication successfully, starting with one that was effective will, in many cases, provide the best outcome.

Conversely, if a patient says he or she has tried a medication but it did not work, get more information about when, for what indication,

Table 7.2 ■ *Common Opioid Medications*

Common Opioid Medications–Short acting			
Medication name	*Generic name/ combination name*	*Usual starting dose–Adults*	*Maximum dose*
codeine	Tylenol #3	30 to 60 milligrams by mouth every 4-6 hours	12 tablets in a 24 hour period Limited by acetaminophen–available as an elixir
hydrocodone	Lortab Vicodin	5 to 10 milligrams by mouth every 4-6 hours 5 to 10 milligrams by mouth every 6 hours	Limited by acetaminophen dose
oxycodone	Percocet	5 milligrams every 6 hours	Limited by acetaminophen dose
tramadol	Ultram Ultracet	25 milligrams by mouth in AM	Maximum 400 milligrams per day Limited by acetaminophen dose
tapentadol	Nucynta	50, 75, or 100 milligrams every 4-6 hours	No more than 700 milligrams on day 1 and thereafter 600 mg maximum
oxymorphone	Opana	10-20 milligrams by mouth every 4 to 6 hours	
hydromorphone	Dilaudid	2 to 4 milligrams by mouth every 4 to 6 hours	Limited only by adverse side effects such as respiratory depression, sedation, nausea

(Continued)

Table 7.2 ■ *(Cont.) Common Opioid Medications*

		Common Opioid Medications–Short acting	
Medication name	*Generic name/ combination name*	*Usual starting dose–Adults*	*Maximum dose*
morphine	Morphine immediate release-MSIR	5 to 15 milligrams by mouth every 4 hours	Limited by adverse side effects such as respiratory depression, sedation, nausea
	Roxanol	5 to 30 milligrams by mouth every 4 hours	
methadone	Dolophine	2.5 to 10 milligrams by mouth every 3 to 4 hours	Extreme care with dosing and medication initiation Half life ranges from 12 to 150 hours

* Acetaminophen dose should be limited to 4000 milligrams per day
Medication information taken from *Nursing 2010 Drug Handbook* and *Opioid Analgesia*, Fine & Portnoy, 2007, and APS, 2008

Common Opioid Medications–Extended Release

* Not intended to be crushed, chewed, or used when alcohol is being ingested

** For use with opioid tolerant patients on a schedule basis–not prn

Medication	*Generic name*	*Usual starting dose*	*Maximum dose*
morphine	Oramorph SR		
	Kadian	20 milligrams every 12 hours or 40 milligrams once daily	
	Avinza	20-30 milligrams by mouth daily	
	MsContin	15 or 30 milligrams every 12 hours	

oxycodone	Oxycontin	10 milligrams every 12 hours	
oxymorphone	Opana ER	5 milligrams every 12 hours	
tramadol	Ultram ER	100 milligrams once daily	300 milligrams per day
dilaudid	Exalgo	8 milligrams to 64 milligrams daily converted from current opioid doses using Exalgo conversion equivalents–give 50% of converted daily dose	
morphine sulfate with naltrexone	Embeda	Convert the patient's total daily dose of current opioid and rescue dose by 50% when initiating therapy–dose every 12 hours	

Medication information taken from *Nursing 2010 Drug Handbook* and *Opioid Analgesia*, Fine & Portnoy, 2007, APS, 2008, and PI for Exalgo, Embeda and Nucynta
In order to be considered opioid tolerant the patients should be taking at least 60 milligrams of oral morphine per day or 25 micrograms of fentanyl patch per hour, 30 milligrams of oxycodone per day
8 milligrams of oral hydromorphone per day, 25 milligrams of oral oxymorphone per day for a week or longer
Source: D'Arcy, Y., & Bruckenthal, P. (2011). *Safe opioid prescribing for nurse practitioners*. New York: Oxford University Press.

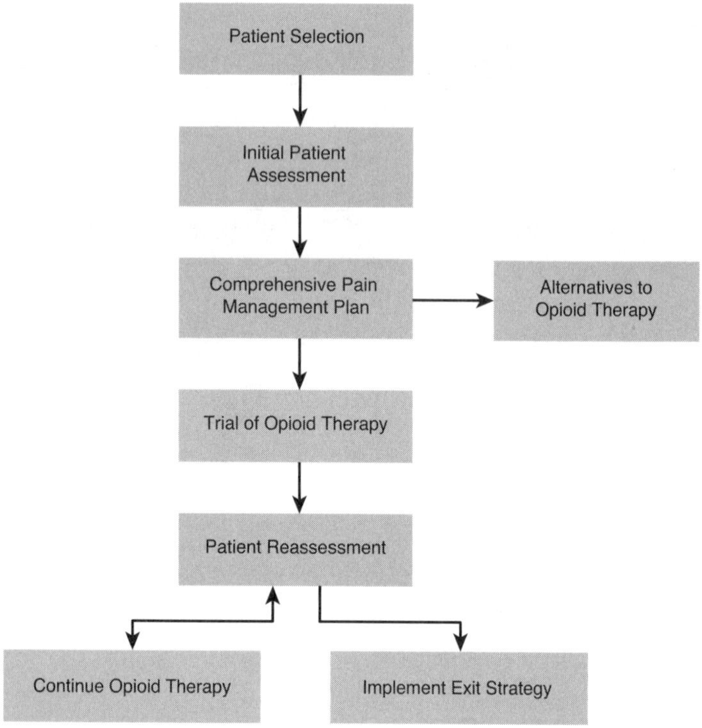

Figure 7.2 ■ Algorithm for opioid treatment of chronic pain

and what doses were tried. In many cases, patients with chronic pain have been underdosed with medications, and they then believe the medications are "not working" or are ineffective. If the correct dose of medication had been provided, the medication could have provided good pain relief. It is always wise to revisit the use of a medication that has been underdosed by using appropriate doses for treating pain unless there are side effects that would contraindicate the use of the drug (Figure 7. 2).

Opioids in the Older Patient

Older patients have a large number of conditions, such as osteoarthritis and other painful comorbidities. Choosing a medication to treat acute pain in these patients is more of a challenge. The myth that older patients do not tolerate pain medications is just that, a myth. Older patients can even use opioid medication with good results if careful dosing and titration takes place.

The American Geriatrics Society (AGS) has released a new set of pain management guidelines for persistent pain in older patients (2009). These new guidelines indicate that opioids are an option for the older patient when moderate to severe pain is present.

For older patients, pain is experienced in the same way, but aging can change the way the nervous system perceives the pain and transmission may be altered (Huffman & Kunik, 2000; McLennon, 2005). Aging can also change the way the older patient's body processes pain medications and can increase the potential for adverse effects. Some of the reasons an older patient may experience adverse effects include the following:

- Muscle-to-fat ratios change as patients age, causing the body fat composition to be altered.
- Poor nutrition can decrease protein stores, which in turn, can decrease the binding ability of some medications.
- Because of the changes in the protein-binding mechanisms, drugs may need to compete for binding sites, making one or more of the patient's medications ineffective.
- Aging affects the physiologic functions of metabolism, absorption, medication clearance (including a slowed GI motility), decreased cardiac output, and decreased glomerular filtration rate.
- Baseline changes in sensory and cognitive perception, such as sedation or confusion, can be an increased risk for some patients.
- Drug excretion and elimination are reduced by 10% for each decade after 40 years of age because of decreased renal function (Bruckenthal & D'Arcy, 2007; D'Arcy, 2009b; Horgas et al., 2003).

The old adage of starting low and going slow still applies to starting opioid therapy in older adults. Older patients are not all the same and bodies age in different ways. Using conservative doses and monitoring the patient carefully for side effects can help ensure that opioids are providing optimal pain relief while also being used safely.

Tips for Starting Analgesic Medication in the Older Patient

Because the older patient has pain needs and requires more monitoring of dosing and adverse effects, starting new medications can be somewhat complicated. Recommendations for pain medications for the older adult (AGS, 2002; 2009) include the following:

- Decrease acetaminophen dose if the patient has a history of alcohol use/abuse or liver or renal impairment. The maximum daily dose should be decreased from 4 g per day by 50% to 75% or not used at all.
- Reduce beginning opioid doses by 25% to 50% to decrease the potential for oversedation.
- Scheduling medication may provide better pain relief and reduce the likelihood of needing increased doses for uncontrolled pain.
- Monitor older adults being started on opioid therapy daily if not more frequently because organ impairment may decrease the elimination of the medication.
- Avoid the use of the following medications because of unwanted side effects and/or toxic metabolites: meperidine, propoxyphene, pentazocine, indomethacin, and amitriptyline (McLennon, 2005).

Treating the Side Effects of Opioid Treatment

All opioids have the potential for side effects. There is no magic opioid or pain medication that does not have the potential for constipation, sedation, or pruritus. Opioids can be used in the presence of side effects, but treatment options to control the unwanted effects or dose reductions to minimize the side effects should be used. One important concept to remember here is that adding a medication that is sedating, such as promethazine, can potentiate sedation from an opioid. Before deciding that an opioid is too sedating, look at all sedating medications that are being used concomitantly and try to minimize the use of additional sedating agents.

Constipation

Constipation is a common side effect of opioid use. It is the one effect to which the patient will not become tolerant. Every patient who is prescribed an opioid should have a laxative of some type. Stool softeners are also used to ease bowel movement. Stimulant laxatives are used to counteract the constipation. Combination stool softener/laxatives are available over the counter in most drugstores. Recommended types of laxatives include the following:

- Senna or Senna with stool softener—increases bowel motility
- bisacodyl—increases bowel motility
- lactulose—osmotic laxative
- sorbitol—osmotic laxative; easily found in Sorbee candies
- methylnaltrexone (Relistor)—approved for opioid-induced constipation for patients with advanced illness or palliative care; subcutaneous injectable (APS, 2008)

Sedation

Patients may become sedated when opioids are first started, but most become tolerant to the effect within a period of 2 weeks or less. If sedation persists or reaches high levels, dose adjustments should be made so that serious oversedation does not occur. Sedation occurs most commonly at the beginning of opioid therapy (D'Arcy, 2007). Patients should be monitored for sedating effects of the opioid and additive sedating effects from medications such as antiemetics, sedatives, antihistamines, muscle relaxants, sleeping medications, benzodiazepines, and so forth.

To counteract sedation, stimulants such as caffeine, dextroamphetamine, methylphenidate, or modafinil can be used. The sedating medications listed previously are most commonly used for patients with chronic cancer pain. Most patients adjust to the sedating effects of opioids within a few weeks at the longest, but the use of caffeine can be recommended for almost any patient.

In acute care, oxygen monitoring or capnography can be used to monitor sedation that could lead to respiratory depression. When giving opioids to postoperative patients, it is wise to monitor the use of other sedating medications with patients who are using opioids for postoperative pain control.

Pruritus (Itching)

Some patients who started on opioids or are taking high doses of opioids may develop pruritus, commonly known as itching. It was thought to be the result of a histamine release, and it is not an indication of a true allergy. Current thinking indicates that it may have its source in an unknown cerebral function. The most common way to counteract the itching is to use an antihistamine such as diphenhydramine (Benadryl). If the itching persists, changing to another opioid may reduce or eliminate this effect. For postoperative patients on PCA and epidurals, the use of small doses of Nubain 2.5 mg IV, a mixed agonist-antagonist medication, is an *off-label* use for treating pruritus.

Delirium/Confusion

Delirium can be caused by opioids, and it is usually a temporary state. Many patients, especially older ones, become confused when they are moved from their usual living situation and put into a new situation or have surgery and start opioids. For patients with chronic pain, the incidence of confusion or delirium should be much less. If the patient becomes delirious, changing the opioid, reducing the dose, or stopping the opioid may provide the needed intervention. Some opioids, such as morphine, have a higher profile for confusion. Changing to another medication, such as low-dose Dilaudid, may provide adequate pain relief and lessen the potential for confusion.

Nausea and Vomiting

Opioids have a high profile for nausea and vomiting. For most opioids, taking the medication with a small amount of food or milk will help to reduce the effect. If the nausea and vomiting do not resolve, using an antiemetic regularly until the effect abates is the best option. Because all antiemetics are sedating, there will be an additive sedating effect when the medications are combined. Recommended antiemetics include the following:

- ondansetron
- Phenergan[2]
- Reglan
- meclizine or cyclizine, for motion-induced nausea
- scopolamine patches, for severe cases (APS, 2008)

---

[2] Phenergan should be used with caution with IV administration. This medication can cause tissue necrosis.

Case Study

Sharon P., 32 years old, is admitted after a fall from a ladder. She has a broken femur, two broken ribs, and a pelvic fracture. There is a suspicion that she has two compression fractures in her lumbar spine, but she has refused to go for an MRI. She complains of pain repeatedly. She will not move for the physical therapist and tells you that the pain is too severe to do anything but stay in one position in bed. She has been told about the need for moving once the surgery was done to repair her femur. She says she can't use the incentive spirometer, and she just feels the pain is too much to bear. She always rates it at 10/10. She has been using a Dilaudid PCA and has 250 attempts and 61 injections, and her dose has not been increased since the PCA was first set up 3 days ago.

How can you impress on Sharon that even though she has pain, she will need to move? How will you improve her pain control?

Questions to Consider

1. What can you add to the medication regimen that will improve the pain relief: NSAIDs, acetaminophen, coanalgesics, or will you change the opioid?
2. Does Sharon have realistic expectations for pain relief?
3. If Sharon has a chronic pain condition, will it color the way she reacts when she has acute pain?
4. Can you start Sharon on an ER pain medication?
5. What types of interventional pain options could you use to improve Sharon's pain?

REFERENCES

Adams, M., & Abdieh, H. (2004). Pharmokinetics and dose-proportionality of oxymorphone extended rclease and its metabolites: Results of a randomized crossover study. *Pharmacotherapy, 24*(4), 468–476.

Adams, M., Pienazek, H., Gammatoni, A., & Abdieh, H. (2005). Oxymorphone extended release does not affect CVP2C9 or CYP3A4 metabolite pathways. *Journal of Clinical Pharmacology, 45,* 337–345.

American Geriatrics Society. (2002). Persistent pain in the older patient. *Journal of the American Geriatrics Society, 50,* S205–S224.

American Geriatrics Society. (2009). Persistent pain in the older patient. *Journal of the American Geriatrics Society, 57,* 1331–1346.

American Pain Society. (2008). *Principles of analgesic use in the treatment of acute pain and cancer pain.* Glenview, IL: Author.

American Society of Pain Management Nursing. (2010). *Core curriculum for pain management nursing.* Dubuque, IA: Kendall Hunt Publishing

Brukenthal, P., & D'Arcy, Y. (2007). Assessment and management of pain in older adults: A review of the basics. *Topics in Advanced Practice Journal, 7*(1). Retrieved July 13, 2009, from http://www.medscape.com/viewarticle

D'Arcy, Y. (2007). *Pain management: Evidence-based tools and techniques for nursing professionals.* Marblehead, MA: HCPro.

D'Arcy, Y. (2009a). Avoid the dangers of opioid therapy. *American Nurse Today, 4*(5), 18–22.

D'Arcy, Y. (2009b). *Pain in the older adult.* Indianapolis, IN: Sigma Theta Tau.

Fine, P., & Portnoy, R. (2007). *A clinical guide to opioid analgesia.* New York: Vendome Group Health Care.

Holden, J. E., Jeong, Y., & Forrest, J. M. (2005). The endogenous opioid system and clinical pain management. *AACN Clinical Issues, 16*(3), 291–301.

Horgas, A. (2003). Pain management in elderly adults. *Journal of Infusion Nursing, 26*(3), 161–165.

Huffman, J., & Kunik, M. (2000). Assessment and understanding of pain in patients with dementia. *The Gerontologist, 40*(5), 574–581.

Katz, N., McCarberg, B., & Reisner, L. (2007). *Managing chronic pain with opioids in primary care.* Newton, MA: Inflexxion.

Løvlie, R., et al. (2001). Polymorphisms in CYP2D6 duplication-negative individuals with the ultrarapid metabolizer phenotype: A role for the CYP2D6*35 allele in ultrarapid metabolism? *Pharmacogenetics, 11*(1), 45–55.

McLennon, S. M. (2005). Persistent pain management. *National Guidelines Clearinghouse.* Retrieved from www.guideline.gov

Nursing 2010 Drug Handbook. (2009). Philadelphia: Lippincott Williams & Wilkins.

ADDITIONAL RESOURCES

Chou, R., Fanciullo, G., Fine, P., Adler, J., Ballantyne, J., Davies, P., . . . Miaskowski, C. (2009). Opioid treatment guidelines: Clinical guidelines for the use of chronic opioid therapy in chronic noncancer pain. *The Journal of Pain, 10*(2), 113–130.

McCoy, A. W. (n.d.). *Opium: Opium history up to 1858 A.D.* Retrieved from http://opioids.com/opium/history/index.html

Osler, W. (n.d.). *The plant of joy.* Retrieved from http://www.opiates.net/

8

Coanalgesics for Additive Pain Relief

COANALGESICS FOR ACUTE PAIN

Coanalgesics are a varied group of medications that can provide additive pain relief when they are added to nonsteroidal anti-inflammatory drugs (NSAIDs) or opioids (American Pain Society [APS], 2008). They can have independent analgesic activity for some painful complaints, and they can counteract select adverse effects of analgesics (APS, 2008). This group of medications was developed to treat a wide variety of conditions, such as seizures or muscle spasms, and were originally intended for symptom control of the various conditions. However, in many cases, patients reported pain relief when these medications were prescribed for them, leading health care providers to consider their additional application for pain relief.

Although some classes of these medications are not used for acute pain, there are some that can be used effectively, such as muscle relaxants. Some of these medications are being used to treat pain on an *off-label* basis. If pain has been determined to have a neuropathic source, antidepressants, antiseizure medications, or topical medications, such as lidoderm patches, can be trialed to see if there is any definitive benefit for relieving the pain. An example of this type of pain is in a patient who has a large amount of tissue damage from surgery or swelling where nerves are being compressed, causing additional pain.

Medications that are considered to be coanalgesics for pain management include the following:

- Antidepressants
- Anticonvulsants
- Muscle relaxants
- Topical agents
- Cannabinoids
- *N*-methyl-d-aspartate (NMDA) receptor blockers
- Alpha 2-adrenergic agonists
- Benzodiazepines
- Antispasmodic agents
- Stimulants (APS, 2008)

Although these medications were not developed for pain control, they have been used for adjunct pain relief and are found to be effective. For some medications, such as gabapentin (Neurontin), pregabalin (Lyrica), and duloxetine (Cymbalta), the pain application became so prevalent that the manufacturers sought and received Food and Drug Administration (FDA) approval for pain management. Many patients with neuropathic pain benefit greatly from the addition of one or more of these agents to help decrease pain. Because many patients with chronic pain are depressed, the use of antidepressants has improved the quality of pain relief and enhanced sleep for many of these patients.

When the World Health Organization (WHO) ladder was developed with medication choices for pain management (see Chapter 6), the focus was on dividing different types of opioid medications. However, the ladder also includes adjuvant medications, or coanalgesics, on each step of the ladder. The broad classes of these medications are listed, but no specific medications are listed so the choice of coanalgesic is patient dependent (Dalton & Youngblood, 2000).

Trying to group these medications into a single class of coanalgesics is difficult. They all have such different mechanisms of action and application. These medications can enhance the effect of opioids or other medications that are being used for pain relief, or they can stand alone as single-agent pain relievers (APS, 2008). Some of the benefits of using these medications include the following:

- Enhance pain relief
- Allow lower doses of opioids (opioid-sparing effect)
- Manage refractory pain
- Reduce side effects of opioids related to opioid sparing (APS, 2008)

Commonly used coanalgesics include the following:

- acetaminophen (Tylenol)
- ibuprofen (Advil, Nuprin), naproxen (Naprosyn), or naproxen sodium (Aleve)
- celecoxib (Celebrex)
- gabapentin (Neurontin) and pregabalin (Lyrica)
- duloxetine hydrochloride (Cymbalta)
- topical lidocaine (Lidoderm) and capsaicin 8% patch (Qutenza)
- cyclobenzaprine hydrochloride (Flexeril), carisoprodol (Soma), or metaxalone (Skelaxin)
- diazepam (Valium) or alprazolam (Xanax) (APS, 2008)

No matter which medication is selected or combined, each patient's comorbidities need to be assessed and evaluated before adding a new medication to the pain management medication regimen. The following sections of the chapter will discuss different classes of coanalgesic that can be used for additional pain relief.

ANTIDEPRESSANT MEDICATIONS

Antidepressant medications are classed into several different types.

- Tricyclic antidepressants (TCAs)
- Selective serotonin reuptake inhibitors (SSRIs)
- Selective serotonin norepinephrine reuptake inhibitors (SSNRIs)

Antidepressant medications have several different mechanisms of action. The TCAs (Table 8.1), such as amitriptyline (Elavil), inhibit presynaptic uptake of norepinephrine and serotonin, as do the

Table 8.1 ■ *Tricyclic Antidepressants*

Common TCAs	*Starting Dose*	*Effective Dose*
amitriptyline (Elavil)	10–25 mg hs	50–150 mg hs
desipramine (Norpramin)	10–25 mg hs	50–150 mg hs
nortriptyline (Pamelor)	10–25 mg hs	50–150 mg hs

Abbreviations: hs, at bedtime; TCA, tricyclic antidepressants.
Source: From American Pain Society, 2008.

SSNRIs, such as duloxetine (Cymbalta). Other less studied actions for TCAs include a mild opioid action at the mu binding sites, sodium and calcium channel blockade, NMDA site antagonism, and adenosine activity (Lynch & Watson, 2006). The SSRI medications, such as fluoxetine hydrochloride (Prozac), inhibit serotonin at the presynaptic junction site (Ghafoor & St. Marie, 2009). The effect of this inhibition decreases the ability of the pain stimulus to be transmitted higher up the central nervous system (D'Arcy, 2007). These medications are most commonly used as adjunct medication for neuropathic type pain, such as postherpetic neuralgia, painful diabetic neuropathies, and neuropathic syndromes (Lynch & Watson, 2006). They are also a good adjunct in patients with cancer and neuropathic pain when opioids have provided suboptimal pain relief (APS, 2008).

The TCAs were at one time considered to be the first line for treating neuropathic pain such as postherpetic neuralgia or postmastectomy pain syndromes. The starting doses are low, 10 to 25 mg titrated up to 150 mg per day (APS, 2008; Wallace & Statts, 2005). Escalating to higher doses to obtain an additive effect for pain relief should take place every 3 to 7 days (Chen et al., 2004). The pain management doses are lower than the antidepressant doses of 150 to 300 mg per day. Of note, the pain relief action of these medications is independent of any effect on mood (Lynch & Watson, 2006).

A meta-analysis of the TCA medications indicates that TCAs are effective for use in treating neuropathic pain (APS, 2008). Elavil is the best known and most studied of the TCAs. It is also a primary recommendation for the treatment of fibromyalgia pain

(D'Arcy & McCarberg, 2005). Analgesic response is usually seen within 5 to 7 days (APS, 2008). Adverse effects of TCAs include the following:

- Sedation
- Dry mouth
- Constipation
- Urinary retention
- Orthostatic hypotension
- Anticholinergic side effects
- Caution in patients with heart disease, symptomatic prostatic hypertrophy, neurogenic bladder, dementia, and narrow angle glaucoma
- Increased suicide behavior in young adults (Institute for Clinical System Improvement [ICSI], 2007)

These side effects make the medications undesirable for use in the elderly, especially when they are used in combination with opioid analgesics.

Additionally, the TCAs can increase the risk of cardiac arrhythmias in patients with underlying conduction abnormalities. Caution with the use of desipramine hydrochloride (Norpramin) in children where anecdotal reports of sudden death have been reported (APS, 2008). Although these drugs are cheap and readily available, they do have some very significant adverse effects. At the opposite end of the spectrum, they also have the best profile for use in treating neuropathic pain conditions. However, each patient being considered for TCAs should have a thorough assessment for any risk factors, such as cardiac conduction abnormalities. When starting TCA therapy, the current recommendation is to screen all patients older than 40 years with an electrocardiogram (ECG) to evaluate the patients for conduction abnormalities (APS, 2008).

The TCA medications are not recommended for use in elderly patients because of the high incidence of undesirable side effects and the potential for increased fall risk related to early morning orthostatic hypotension (American Geriatrics Society [AGS], 2002; Lynch & Watson, 2006). The biggest benefits of using TCAs for pain relief are improved sleep (Wilson et al., 1997) and the relief of neuropathic pain—pain that is described by patients as burning, shooting, or painful numbness (D'Arcy, 2007).

When caring for a patient who is taking TCAs as adjuvant pain medication, health care providers should be aware of the potential for early morning orthostatic hypotension and caution patients to sit on the side of the bed for a few minutes before trying to stand. Some patients complain of sleepiness with these medications, and if this is problematic, the patient should be instructed to take the medication earlier in the evening rather than at bedtime, to decrease the early morning sedation that can be experienced. For elderly men, urinary retention can be problematic and urinary status should be carefully checked. For the dry mouth associated with TCA use, hard candies or gum can ease the dry feeling.

Patients should always be told the rationale for prescribing an antidepressant medication for pain so they are comfortable taking the medication. The onset of analgesic effect may take up to 2 weeks, and patients should be encouraged to extend a trial of these medications to this period to see if analgesia occurs.

Of all three groups of antidepressants, the SSRI group (Table 8.2) has the poorest profile for pain relief (APS, 2006). When compared with placebo, these medications did not have any significant advantage for pain relief. Given the lack of efficacy for pain relief in these medications and the profile of side effects (e.g., sexual dysfunction, anxiety, sleep disorder, and headache), the SSRIs are not the medications that should be given unless there is a specific indication for use. The recommended use for this group of medications is for patients who have concurrent depression, anxiety, or insomnia (APS, 2008).

Table 8.2 ■ *Selective Serotonin Reuptake Inhibitors*

	Starting Dose	*Effective Dose*
paroxetine (Paxil)	10–20 mg daily	20–40 mg daily
citalopram (Celexa)	10–20 mg daily	20–40 mg daily

Source: From American Pain Society, 2008.

The pain relief mechanism of the SNRI group of antidepressants (Table 8.3) is the inhibition of serotonin and norepinephrine at therapeutic doses (APS, 2008). The SNRI medications do not have the same anticholinergic side effect profile as TCA medications. They are effective for various neuropathic pain conditions, such as diabetic neuropathy, postherpetic neuralgia, and atypical facial pain (Lynch & Watson, 2006). Venlafaxine (Effexor) has shown an effect on hyperalgesia and allodynia, both preventing the occurrence of and decreasing pain (APS, 2008; Wallace & Staats, 2005). Effective doses for venlafaxine for pain relief range from 150 to 225 mg, with a starting dose of 37.5 mg.

Duloxetine (Cymbalta) has received FDA approval for treating painful diabetic neuropathy (PDN). For duloxetine, the starting dose of 20 mg daily may decrease the incidence of side effects with pain relief being experienced at a dose range from 60 to 120 mg daily. Careful titration of the medications and slow dose increases will help decrease some of the side effects, such as somnolence, nausea, and sweating. There have been no identified increased cardiovascular risks associated with the use of duloxetine (APS, 2008).

There are some drawbacks with both venlafaxine and duloxetine. There is an increased risk of suicidal ideation and behavior in children and adolescents with major depressive disorders, and neither is approved for pediatric patients. Care should also be taken with patients who have liver disease or use alcohol consistently (Cymbalta package insert, prescribing information; Nurse Practitioner Prescribing reference, Winter 2006–2007, available at www.PrescribingReference.com). There is also the potential for the development of sick serotonin syndrome, which occurs when patients taking SNRI medications take other medications that affect serotonin production, such as SSRI medications.

Table 8.3 ■ *Serotonin and Norepinephrine Reuptake Inhibitors*

	Starting Dose	*Effective Dose*
venlafaxine (Effexor)	37.5 mg daily	150–225 mg daily
duloxetine (Cymbalta)	20 mg daily	60 mg daily

Source: From American Pain Society, 2008.

Cardiac changes are also possible with atrioventricular (AV) block and increases in blood pressure (Lynch & Watson, 2006). Of venlafaxine-treated patients, 5% developed changes on ECG (APS, 2008). As a result, patients who are taking venlafaxine who also have diabetes mellitus, hypertension, or hypercholesterolemia, or are currently smoking should have ECG monitoring while on the antidepressant medication (APS, 2008). Patients who are taking these medications for adjunct pain relief should have regular blood pressure screenings and should be assessed regularly for any signs of cardiac changes. Careful dose tapering should take place when these medications are being discontinued to avoid discontinuation syndrome, insomnia, lethargy, diarrhea, nausea, dizziness, or paresthesia (APS, 2008).

ANTICONVULSANT MEDICATIONS

Anticonvulsants (Table 8.4) are commonly used to treat neuropathic pain of different types, such as postherpetic neuralgia, painful diabetic neuralgia (PDN), and trigeminal neuralgia (APS, 2006). The original premise for use was that if these medications could control the erratic neuronal firing or seizures, it could be applied for controlling neuronal discharge from pain stimuli. Research has shown that this is essentially true, and one of the primary mechanisms of these medications is to reduce neuronal excitability and spontaneous firing of cortical neurons (APS, 2008). When applied to pain management, these

Table 8.4 ■ *Anticonvulsant Medications*

Commonly Used Anticonvulsants	*Starting Dose*	*Effective Dose*
gabapentin (Neurontin)	100–300 mg hs	300–1200 mg tid
pregabalin (Lyrica)	150 mg daily	300–600 mg daily
carbamazepine (Tegretol)	100–200 mg daily	300–800 mg bid
topiramate (Topamax)	25 mg daily	100–200 mg bid
phenytoin (Dilantin)	300 mg hs	100–150 mg tid

Abbreviations: bid, two times a day; hs, at bedtime; tid, three times a day.

drugs are thought to decrease the neuronal firing for neuropathic pain and to decrease neuronal sensitization (APS, 2008).

Anticonvulsant agents are commonly used for treating neuropathic pain. Gabapentin (Neurontin) is one of the medications used to treat a multitude of neuropathic pain syndromes; however, it is particularly effective with postherpetic neuralgia, diabetic neuropathy, phantom limb pain, Guillain-Barré syndrome, neuropathic cancer pain, and acute and chronic spinal cord injury (APS, 2008; ICSI, 2007). Syndromes that do not respond to gabapentin include HIV-related neuropathy and painful peripheral chemotherapy-induced neuropathies (APS, 2008).

Both gabapentin (Neurontin) and pregabalin (Lyrica) act by blocking neuronal calcium channels, the alpha 2-delta subunit specifically reducing the release of glutamate, norepinephrine, and substance P (APS, 2008). Because the drugs are renally excreted, dose reductions are advised for patients with renal impairment. The drawback to gabapentin is the length of time needed to reach effective dose strength; it is only 10% bioavailable. Because medication response is patient dependent, it may take several weeks or months to reach a dose of gabapentin that will provide pain relief. Pregabalin, as an alternate option, can provide a faster response for pain relief because therapeutic doses can be given earlier in the treatment and it has a 90% bioavailability.

For acute pain, gabapentin and pregabalin have demonstrated an opioid-sparing effect of up to 60% when the medications are given preoperatively at doses of 300 to 1200 mg. The drawback is the increased sedation that has also been reported.

The older anticonvulsants, such as phenytoin (Dilantin), have not been studied for pain relief as fully as the newer gabapentin medications and thus have only weak evidence for their use as coanalgesic medications for pain. There is a need for further research data. One early meta-analysis (McQuay et al., 1995, in APS, 2008) determined that four anticonvulsants, including phenytoin, carbamazepine (Tegretol), clonazepam (Klonopin), and valproate (Depacon), were effective for relieving the pain of trigeminal neuralgia, diabetic neuropathy, and migraine prophylaxis. Given the high profile for serious adverse side effects, the new gabapentin medications are indicated as first line for treating neuropathic pain (APS, 2008).

One of the major drawbacks to anticonvulsant medications is their high profile for adverse side effects. These include the following:

- Somnolence
- Dizziness
- Fatigue
- Nausea
- Edema
- Weight gain
- Stevens-Johnson syndrome
- Increased risk of suicidal behavior or ideation
- Aplastic anemia and agranulocytosis (ICSI, 2007)

The serious nature of the adverse side effects of this class of medications makes it imperative that when starting these medications, a full baseline history is taken from the patient. Careful monitoring is required, and the patients should be instructed to report the occurrence and severity of any adverse effect if it happens.

TOPICAL ANALGESICS

Lidocaine 5% Patch (Lidoderm)

When the patient has a specific tender point or has an area of pain that is limited, it is tempting to use a type of pain relief that will affect only the painful area. The lidocaine patch (5%) is a soft flannel-backed patch with 5% lidocaine that can be applied over the painful area. It has an indication for use with postherpetic neuralgia and has been studied in painful diabetic neuropathy, complex regional pain syndrome, postmastectomy pain, and HIV-related neuropathy (APS, 2008).

The patch is designed to be used for 12 hours on and 12 hours off, although patients have worn the patch for 24 hours with no ill effects (APS, 2008; D'Arcy, 2007). The maximum dose of Lidoderm is up to three patches at one time. The patches should be replaced daily and placed only on intact skin. Active serum levels of lidocaine with patch use are minimal (APS, 2008). Patients tolerate this type of therapy very well and because it is noninvasive, should the patient not like the feeling of the patch or effect, the patch can be easily removed. The only side effect from the Lidoderm patch that has been reported is rare instances of skin irritation at the site of patch application.

Capsaicin Cream (Zostrix)

Capsaicin is a topical cream that can reduce the secretion of substance P at peripheral nerve ending and is derived from hot peppers. It is sold over the counter in two different strengths as Zostrix cream. The neuropathic conditions for which this cream has been most helpful include postmastectomy pain, other peripheral neuropathic conditions, and neck and arthritis pain (APS, 2008).

When the cream is applied, it causes a burning sensation in the application area. Patients should be warned to expect the sensation. Gloves should be used to apply the cream to the painful area; other parts of the body, such as the eyes, should not be touched until all the cream is removed from the hands. This technique requires a dedicated patient who is willing to persevere and apply the cream 3 to 4 times per day for 2 weeks to see if there is any analgesic benefit.

A new 8% capsaicin patch called Qutenza is used for postherpetic neuralgia. It needs to be applied by a health care provider who has been trained in the technique. Local anesthetic is applied over the site of the pain, and the patch is applied for an hour and removed. This form of capsaicin can provide up to 12 weeks of pain relief.

Targeted Analgesic-Diclofenac Epolamine Patch (Flector)

The Flector patch is a nonselective NSAID patch that is applied directly over the site of the pain on intact skin. It is especially useful for strains and sprains. The recommended dose is one patch to the affected area twice a day (Nursing, 2010, 2009). Because this is a new use for NSAIDs, the research support is limited and data on systemic absorption are open to change when clinical usage increases. Currently, the medication has the same black box warning of all nonselective NSAIDs.

There are compounded gels and over-the-counter NSAID gel formulations as well. These can be very effective if used as directed in the prescribed area. However, with continued use and application over large areas, there is an increased potential for systemic absorption. Patients are advised to use the application card supplied with the medication and wear gloves when applying the gel (*Nursing 2010 Drug Handbook*, 2009).

MUSCLE RELAXANTS

Muscle relaxants are a good addition to a pain regimen for conditions, such as low back pain, in which muscle spasms occur regularly. They are also useful for conditions, such as fibromyalgia, for which cyclobenzaprine is considered a first-line option (APS, 2005; D'Arcy & McCarberg, 2005). The group of medications, generically called skeletal muscle relaxants, consists of several different groups of medications: benzodiazepines, sedatives, antihistamines, and other centrally acting medications (Tables 8.5 and 8.6) (APS, 2008).

Although there is no indication that these medications relax skeletal muscles, they are commonly used for spasm and muscle tightness (APS, 2008). After 1 to 2 weeks, the action of the medication shifts to a central activity rather than skeletal muscle activity (APS, 2008). The most common side effect of this group of medica-

Table 8.5 ■ *Skeletal Muscle Relaxants*

	Starting Dose	*Effective Dose*
cyclobenzaprine (Fexeril)	5 mg tid	10–20 mg tid
carisoprodol (Soma)	350 mg hs-tid	350 mg tid-qid
orphenadrine (Norflex)	100 mg bid	100 mg bid
tizanidine (Zanaflex)	2 mg hs	Variable
metaxalone (Skelaxin)	400 mg tid-qid	800 mg tid-qid
methocarbamol (Robaxin)	500 mg qid	500–750 mg qid

Abbreviations: bid, twice daily; hs, at bedtime; tid, three times a day; qid, four times a day.
Source: From American Pain Society, 2008.

Table 8.6 ■ *Other Types of Relaxants*

antispasmodic (Baclofen)	5 mg tid	10–20 mg tid
benzodiazepine (Diazepam)	1 mg bid	2–10 mg bid-qid

Abbreviations: bid, two times a day; qid, four times a day; tid, three times a day.
Source: From American Pain Society, 2008.

tions is sedation. If they are being use concomitantly with opioid analgesic, the sedative effect is cumulative. There is the potential for abuse in patients who are predisposed to this problem, so intermittent or short-term use is advised.

OTHER TYPES OF COANALGESICS

There are various other medications that can be used as coanalgesics, ranging from cannabinoids, such as dronabinol, which are recommended for neuropathic pain from multiple sclerosis, to NMDA receptor blockers, such as ketamine, dextromethorphan (Benylin, Robitussin), and amantadine (Symmetrel), used for centrally mediated neuropathic pain and hyperalgesia. These agents are not recommended for first- or second-line use, but rather for patients who have failed all other attempts for pain relief. They have a high profile for little research support and lean more on anecdotal and single study support.

These medications also have a high profile for significant adverse side effects. Dronabinol use can cause cognitive impairment, psychosis, and sedation (APS, 2008).

The NMDA receptor blockers have significant adverse side effects, such as ketamine-induced hallucinations, memory problems, and abuse potential; amantadine and dextromethorphan have less severe side effects, such as dizziness, insomnia, and nausea (*Nursing 2010 Drug Handbook*, 2009).

When considering the use of a coanalgesic, the health care provider needs to fully assess the patient and consider all the comorbidities and potential drug-drug interactions. The use of these medications is highly individualized, and doses may vary according to the patient's ability to tolerate the medications. Starting a lower dose and escalating slowly can help reduce the seriousness of the side effects. Because analgesic effect can take time to become apparent, patients should be encouraged to use these medications for at least 2 weeks before deciding if they are not effective for pain relief.

Case Study

John C. is an 86-year-old patient who is admitted with intractable pain after a herpes zoster infection. He is rolling in the bed when you see him, moaning and crying out. He pleads with you, "Please, please make this pain stop." When you examine the painful area, it is the site of a healed rash across the thorax on one side. His family tells you he has not slept in weeks, and not one of the pain medications he has used works. He can't even stand to have clothes touch his skin so he has stopped wearing a shirt. His current pain medications are hydrocodone (Vicodin) and ibuprofen.

The pain is 10/10 in intensity. How will you manage his pain?

Questions to Consider

1. What type of opioids will you use, more orals, IV, patient-controlled analgesia (PCA), or epidural?
2. What is the condition of pain with his clothes touching him called?
3. What types of coanalgesics can you use?
4. Would an interventional pain management option work for John?
5. Would you consider using Qutenza?

REFERENCES

American Geriatrics Society Panel on Persistent Pain in Older Persons. (2002, 2009). The management of persistent pain in older persons. *Journal of the American Geriatrics Society, 50*, S205–S224.

American Pain Society. (2006). *Pain control in the primary care setting.* Glenview, IL: Author.

American Pain Society. (2008). *Principles of analgesic use in the treatment of acute and cancer pain*. Glenview, IL: Author.

Chen, H., Lamer, T. J., Rho, R. H., Marshall, K. A., Sitzman, B. T., Ghazi, S. M., & Brewer, R. P. (2004). Contemporary management of neuropathic pain for the primary care physician. *Mayo Clinic Proceedings, 79*(12), 1533–1545.

Dalton, J. A., & Youngblood, R. (2000). Clinical application of the World Health Organization analgesic ladder. *Journal of Intravenous Nursing, 23*(2), 118–124.

D'Arcy, Y., & McCarberg, B. (2005). New fibromyalgia pain management recommendations. *The Journal for Nurse Practitioners, 1*(4), 218–225.

D'Arcy, Y. (2007). *Pain management: Evidence-based tools and techniques for nursing professionals.* Marblehead, MA: HCPro.

Ghafoor, V., & St. Marie, B. (2009). *Overview of pharmacology in core curriculum for pain management nursing.* Indianapolis, IN: Kendall Publications.

Institute for Clinical System Improvement. (2007). *Assessment and management of chronic pain*. Bloomington, MN: Author.

Lynch, M. E., & Watson, C. P. N. (2006). The pharmacotherapy of chronic pain: A review. *Pain Research & Management, 11*(1), 11–38.

Nursing 2010 Drug Handbook. (2009). Philadelphia, PA: Lippincott Williams & Wilkins.

Wallace, M. S., & Staats, P. S. (2005). *Pain medicine and management.* New York: McGraw-Hill.

Wilson, P., Caplan, R., Connis, R., Gilbert, H., Grigsby, E., Haddox, D., . . . Simon, D. (1997). Practice guidelines for chronic pain management: A report by the American Society of Anesthesiologists Task Force on Pain Management, Chronic Pain Section. *Anesthesiology, 86*(4), 995–1004.

9

The Effect of Opioid Polymorphisms and Patient Response to Medications

PATIENT DIFFERENCES IN PAIN MANAGEMENT

One of the newest pieces of pain management research is focused on the effect of the patient's gender and genetic makeup on pain medication binding and utilization. For many years, there has been a speculation by clinicians as to why some patients responded well to small doses of opioids and got excellent pain relief, whereas other patients required large doses to get even minimal pain relief. Patients with specific types of surgery were compared, and the individual differences were striking. The answer being not all patients with a colon resection, hysterectomy, or prostate surgery respond to pain medications in the same way. Individualization is needed.

For many years, a patient was considered to be drug seeking if large doses of medication were required to control pain. Patients were considered to be exemplary if they could manage pain relief with small amounts of medication. Little concern was given to the individual differences that all patients bring to the pain management setting. Because little was known about how genetics, sex, gender, and pain were related, the patient often felt that he or she was being blamed for any lack of success with pain management regimens.

Today, we know that pain relief is not a single entity based on putting the right medication into the right patient, but one that is more reliant on patient genetics and pathophysiology. As noted in Chapter 7, not all patients can use certain pain medications, such as codeine, because they lack the liver enzyme needed to convert the codeine to morphine, the active form. As research progresses, findings indicate that there are many genetic factors that play an important role in how pain medications work for the individual patient.

Patients with chronic pain also have a changed response to subsequent pain stimulus because the repeated pain stimuli cause the nervous system to modify its function to react more comprehensively. This is called *neuronal plasticity* (Rowbotham, Kidd, & Porreca, 2006). Neuronal plasticity can result in the phenomenon called peripheral sensitization, where nociception in peripheral neurons is heightened, and pain stimuli are felt to be more severe than is indicated by the stimulus. As the pain stimuli continues, pain-facilitating substances, such as cytokines and substance P, are recruited to the area, leading to increased pain sensation, inflammation, and the development of hyperalgesia and allodynia.

Wind-up is another physiologic change that occurs when the pain response in the central nervous system is activated as a result of the continued peripheral pain input. As the pain continues, the phenomenon called wind-up allows the patient to experience pain that is more intense, prolonged, and much more difficult to treat. With wind-up, the *N*-methyl-d-aspartate (NMDA) receptors are activated and help accelerate and increase the intensity of the pain stimuli. Examples of diseases in which wind-up becomes very problematic are osteoarthritis and rheumatoid arthritis (Rowbotham et al., 2006).

Clinical Pearl

- Neuronal plasticity: Ability of the nervous system to change or alter its function, caused by continued nociceptive input increasing pain intensity and can cause peripheral sensitization
- Wind-up: Enhanced response to pain stimulus, produced by prolonged pain input causing activation of the pain response in the central nervous system

Over the years, as more has become known about the effect of pain, how pain is processed, and how pain response is formulated, there is a rich area of research that has now begun to look at what the role of genetics, gender, and race may be in how pain is perceived and processed. Although the area is still very new, the information in this chapter will provide some early insight into what is known about the differences we cannot control and how that can affect pain modulation and medication effectiveness.

Gender and Pain

Since the early Biblical days of Adam and Eve, who were doomed to experience physical suffering because of their errors in judgment, pain has become a topic of great discussion. How pain is perceived, produced, why it occurs, and what treatment options are effective has been discussed by both academics and average citizens. One topic that continues to be debated is the question of differences in pain sensation between men and women: does it exist, and if so, what is causing these suspected differences? Recent research into the difference between men and women's pain has provided some interesting information and created a need for much more research on the topic.

Do men and women experience pain differently? Yes, they do as a result of their hormonal variation and differences in pain pathway activation when a pain stimulus is presented for interpretation. Are there differences in the way that men and women respond to pain medications? Again, the answer is yes, for various reasons. Some of these differences include the following:

- Specific, different pain pathways for men and women
- Differences in the way pain is processed
- Effect of sex hormones
- Differences in response to opioid medications
- Differences in the threshold and tolerance for pain (Wilson, 2006)

For many years, women were eliminated from research because it was thought that there was an estrogenic effect on pain that would skew research results. Another concern was that estrogen levels in women fluctuated during menstrual cycles and might cause data to be skewed, depending on the time of the month. Because of these suspicions, most of the early research in breast cancer was done with male subjects. Animal studies on pain were performed with desexed animals, hoping to avoid any hormonal effect on the study results. Now, research focuses on these differences and uses them to advantage, such as research into the causes and treatment options for menstrual migraines.

There are some pain conditions that are more specific to women than men. Examples of these syndromes include the following:

- Fibromyalgia
- Temporomandibular joint (TMJ) pain
- Phantom breast pain
- Postmastectomy pain syndrome
- Menstrually related migraine
- Irritable bowel syndrome (IBS)
- Interstitial cystitis
- Vulvodynia

In a study to compare the analgesic effect of morphine in both men and women, three important conclusions were derived.

- Morphine is more potent in women than men.
- The onset and offset of morphine are slower in women than in men.
- Plasma concentrations of both the active drug and two metabolites were identical for both sexes (Dahan, Kest, Waxman, & Sarton, 2008).

These findings are particularly important for acute pain and postoperative pain management. Because morphine is considered the gold standard for pain management medication comparison and is commonly used in postoperative pain relief, these differences in potency and onset are important considerations when pain relief is assessed. As an interesting addendum, the sex effect with morphine disappears with older patients, leading to the speculation that hormones have an effect on morphine's ability to pass through the blood-brain barrier (Dahan et al., 2008).

In addition to the differences in morphine with men and women, the side effects from opioid medications tend to have some sex-related relationships. The most common side effects with opioid medications are nausea/vomiting, sedation, cardiovascular effects, and respiratory depression. These differences include the following:

- More nausea/vomiting with women using opioids for postoperative pain control
- Increased risk for opioid-induced respiratory depression in women
- Morphine associated with lower heart rate in women but the development of hypertension in men
- With opioid use, women reported more feelings of euphoria (a high feeling) and reported more instances of dry mouth (Dahan et al., 2008)

Other differences with pain medications were related to differences seen with kappa agonist medications, such as nalbuphine (Nubain), butorphanol (Stadol), and pentazocine (Talwin Nx).

The melanocortin-1 receptor (MC1R) gene has a specific role in modulating a pain pathway that exists only in women. This gene is commonly associated with people who have red hair, fair skin, freckles, and a high predisposition to melanoma (Dahan et al., 2008).

- MCIR was tested by giving pentazocine to both men and women.
- MCIR showed no pain relief in men but pain relief in women who were redheaded and fair skinned.
- The hypothesis is that men and women have separate pain pathways that are created by different genes and neurochemicals (Mogil, 2006)

The study of differences in pain response both physiologically and to pain medications in men and women is a very new area of research. Much more research is needed to confirm these early findings. The early research is promising and points the way to finding the true differences between men and women in both pain response and medication efficacy.

Genetic Response Variability and Opioid Polymorphisms

We already know that genetics plays a big role in the production of eye color, for example. Some people can have variants of blue, green, gray, or brown eyes based on the dominant gene expression in their individual physiology. What we are just learning is that people can also respond to opioids differently based on their genetic makeup.

One of the most promising targets for study is the A118G single nucleotide polymorphism in the mu-opioid receptor (MOR) gene (Janicki et al., 2006; Landau, 2006). Differences in this section of genetic code are hypothesized to create differences in opioid needs and pain relief.

In a research study with patients (n = 74) who were undergoing total knee replacement, patients were genetically profiled by opioid-binding site types. Group 1 was AA homozygous patients who had a genetically efficient morphine metabolism pattern, Group 2 was an AG heterozygous genetic variant, and Group 3 was a GG homozygous nonsensitive genetic variant with reduced or impaired morphine sensitivity. The findings of morphine use via patient-controlled analgesia (PCA) and analgesia in the first 48 hours postoperatively were significantly different for both morphine consumption and pain relief.

- AA used 25 mg of morphine and had good pain relief.
- AG used 25 mg of morphine and had good pain relief.
- GG used 40 mg of morphine and had many more attempts on their PCAs trying to achieve better pain control (Chou et al., 2006).

What does this mean for the clinician? It does explain some of what we see in the clinical setting with variation in patient response to opioids. Some patients may be genetically programmed to have a good, efficient response to morphine, whereas other patients might benefit from another medication that is more suited to their genetic makeup.

In a prospective, observational study with both patients on acute care (n = 101) and patients with chronic noncancer pain (n = 121), the results were somewhat different. The patients were typed as either having A118 MOR (major) or as having variant G118 MOR (minor) alleles. The results of the acute pain of the postoperative group showed no statistically significant difference in pain scores or in morphine consumption in either group (Janicki et al., 2006). The patients with chronic pain did have some differences between the two groups of patients. In the patients with chronic pain group, the carriers of the major allele required significantly higher doses of opioids when compared with the patients with the minor allele (Janicki et al., 2006).

Clinical Pearl

Opioid Polymorphism: Differences in Opioid Effect Based on Genetic Differences

The variation of the study results could be expected. The area of research is so new that not many replications have been performed, and study protocols are widely variant. As more research is done, there should be some consistent findings to illustrate the differences among patient groups, medications, and pain medication delivery systems (e.g., PCA vs. oral).

What does this mean for clinicians? The results of the studies do seem to indicate that genetic differences can cause a patient to need more morphine to control pain. They do seem to indicate that the patients with the major gene expression (A118 MOR) had a higher need for pain medication as compared with the minor allele group (G118 MOR) if the pain was chronic. However, do genetics account for all the differences? In reality, morphine use on a PCA can be a somewhat unreliable way to measure a patient's desire for using morphine for pain relief, need for medication, fear of addiction, or occurrence of side effects. If a patient is nauseated, they may defer using the PCA because the pain is less burdensome than the nausea.

The biggest indication from these very basic and early studies is that there is a need for more research to better define and confirm the findings of the previous studies. There is an element of excitement here that the findings could really lead to a breakthrough about why patients have such variation in response to opioids and could possibly lead to the creation of a way to predetermine what type of medication or dose would be best for any patient. Only more research can prove or disprove these early studies and determine if we will ever be able to know what pain medication will give which patient the best pain relief.

OPIOID ROTATION AND EQUIANALGESIA

Many endogenous and exogenous substances, including opioids, bind to specific sites in the patient's body. Early research identified the site for opioids binding as the mu-receptor and there followed groups of studies to determine just how the binding was accomplished. As research progressed, various differences in the opioid receptors were discovered, and current research indicates that there are more than 40 different subtypes at the mu-receptor sites (Pasternak, 2005).

Because of these variations, it is common to try one medication, have it fail, try another medication and have it work well to relieve the patient's pain. The ability of the medication to relieve pain is truly a function of the patient's genetics and the binding ability of the medication. If the patient's best binding potential is set up for morphine, giving the patient fentanyl (Sublimaze) for pain will result in poorer outcomes and diminished pain relief.

As the binding sites become accustomed to certain pain medications, the pain relief response can be decreased. These are patients who report less effective pain relief with one medication after dose escalations and interval adjustment. As the doses go up, the side effect profile becomes more burdensome, so little is gained in the way of pain relief and side effects increase. In these cases, a technique called opioid rotation can help increase pain relief and decrease side effects, all at lower doses of a new medication.

Opioid rotation is the clinical practice of substituting one strong opioid for another strong opioid in an attempt to account for incomplete cross-tolerance and achieve a better balance between pain relief and side effects (Quigley, 2004). Another way to describe the rotation effect is switching opioids from one to another when treatment-limiting toxicity establishes poor responsiveness (Indelicato & Portnoy, 2002). Simplistically, the opioid receptor gets a little tired and overly accustomed to seeing one drug all the time, and it will perk up and accept (bind to) a new drug more efficiently, thereby providing a higher level of pain relief with fewer side effects.

Which patients are candidates for opioid rotation? Chronic cancer patients who are heavily opioid dependent are excellent candidates for opioid rotation and may have a group of medications that they rotate through regularly. Chronic pain patients who have taken opioids for an extended period are also very good candidates for opioid rotation. This phenomenon was first seen in chronic pain patients when their opioid use had continued over the course of several years (Indelicato & Portnoy, 2002).

What do these patients look like clinically? These are the patients who complain of poor pain relief and even though you escalate the dose, they continue to complain of pain at the same level with no improvement. In addition, as the doses continue to increase, there is a potential for side effects such as nausea or pruritis, or other unwanted side effects. The risk-benefit ratio of medication use is reached, and further dose escalation would not be useful.

In a study with patients who had cancer (n = 164), changes in opioid medication were tracked. In this patient group, 56% of the patients required opioid rotation related to side effects and ineffective pain relief. The medications being manipulated in this study were morphine, hydromorphone, methadone, fentanyl, and oxycodone (Walsh et al., 2004).

The end result of opioid rotation is improved pain relief with a lower dose of medication. To perform an opioid rotation, there are several steps to follow. Using the equianalgesic table (Table 7.1 in Chapter 7), convert your old medication dose to a new equianalgesic dose of the new medication. Equianalgesia just means equal in analgesic strength. The warning with using these tables is to remember that the doses were set in single dose studies with opioid-naïve patients in acute care settings (Pasternak, 2005). They do not fully capture medication differences over the long term and cannot account for patient variability.

To perform the opioid rotation, calculate the correct conversion of the medication using the table and then decrease the new dose by 25% to 50% and offer adequate breakthrough medication (Indelicato & Portnoy, 2002). The reduction in dose is needed because of the anticipated incomplete cross-tolerance (caused by the differences in mu-receptor and binding) that leads to greater effect and increased side effects if the dose were converted at full strength (D'Arcy, 2009).

Additionally, the individual patient needs to be considered, along with comorbidities and age range (Indelicato & Portnoy, 2002).

Opioid Rotation Conversion Example

Original medication: MS-Contin

MS-Contin 120 mg twice per day with morphine sulfate immediate release (MSIR) 30 mg every 4 hours as needed for pain

New medication: Oxycontin

MS-Contin 120 mg twice per day (240 mg/day) is equal to Oxycontin 80 mg twice per day (160 mg/day)

MSIR 30 mg is equal to oxycodone 20 mg every 4 hours

Decrease the new dose by 25% to 50%

25% = Oxycontin 60 mg twice per day with 15 mg oxycodone every 4 hours for breakthrough

50% = Oxycontin 40 mg twice per day with 10 mg of oxycodone every 4 hours for breakthrough

There is no hard and fast rule about using morphine for breakthrough with extended-release morphine or oxycodone with Oxycontin, but the illustration helps to show an additional conversion by also including the breakthrough option. As a prescriber, you can choose to mix and match morphine with other drugs and vice versa. The key here is to choose medications that the patient has not seen in awhile and to monitor the effect closely, so that you can see if the change has made any difference. If you choose to go with the conservative option, 50%, you can always increase the new medication up to the 25% reduction to improve pain relief if the patient starts to have increased pain. If the patient is someone who can tolerate a bigger dose, considering previous medication history, age, and comorbidities, the 25% option may work best. Always offer adequate breakthrough medication so the patient can more easily convert to the new medication regimen and retain pain control.

OTHER FACTORS

There are other factors that contribute to the use and response to opioids in the body that can also affect pain management outcomes. The liver has a group of enzymes that affect how medications are metabolized or inactivated, or provide a diminished or exaggerated response. The CYP 450 system in the liver transforms some opioids to usable metabolites. If this system is impaired or inactivated by another medication, the opioid effect will be directly affected.

Some patients have different metabolism profiles for medication utilization. If the patient has a rapid or ultrarapid medication metabolism, medication will be used quickly. These are the patients who tell you that a standard dose of opioid medication just does not last long enough. In the medication section, the warning for codeine was highlighted for rapid metabolizers because several incidents of morphine overdose were detected in infants who were nursing from mothers who had taken codeine and rapidly metabolized the codeine to morphine (see Chapter 7, Opioid Medications).

Conversely, at the other end of the spectrum, patients who metabolize medication slowly are at risk for increased effects of opioids with repeated doses. These are the patients who may tell you a small dose of opioid medication lasts a long period, or they request low-dose opioids because they report being "sensitive" to opioids. These patients may also have a higher profile for oversedation, nausea/vomiting, and so forth because the medication stays in their system for a longer period.

No matter what aspect of genetic variability you encounter in clinical practice, there are options to counteract the effect. Switching medications, trying different types of medications, adding in coanalgesics, or complementary methods may increase the potential for optimal pain relief. This is one area where pain management is truly an art and science, and in this case, the science is helping to facilitate the chances of finding the right medication for the individual patient.

Case Study

Sally J. is a 25-year-old patient who is in labor. She is fair skinned and red headed. She tells you that no pain medications ever work for her. Even if she does take pain medication, it never lasts for very long. She gets very nauseated and vomits with most opioid pain medication. She does not want an epidural and would like to try to deliver the baby naturally. As her labor progresses, Sally begins to ask for pain medication. She can't tell you what has worked for her. How will you manage her labor pain?

Questions to Consider

1. Do you suspect that Sally's genetic profile would indicate she has some difficulty with morphine metabolism?
2. What does being a fair-skinned, redheaded woman have to do with Sally's pain management?
3. Does Sally's gender have a role in her lack of pain relief with opioids?
4. How would you classify Sally's opioid metabolism?
5. What kind of nonopioids would you suggest: NSAIDs, APAP, anticonvulsants, antidepressants, and so forth?
6. Would adding a complementary method to her pain management regimen be helpful? What would you suggest for a patient in labor?

REFERENCES

American Pain Society. (2008). *Principles of analgesic use in the treatment of acute pain and cancer pain* (6th ed.). Glenview, IL: Author.

Chou, W. Y., Yang, L. C., Lu, H. F., Ko, J. Y., Wang, C. H., Lin, S. H., & Hsu, C. J. (2006). Association of μ-opioid receptor gene polymorphism (A118G) with variations in morphine consumption for analgesia after total knee arthroplasty. *Acta Anaesthesiologica Scandinavica, 50*(7), 787–792.

Dahan, A., Kest, B., Waxman, A. R., & Sarton, E. (2008). Sex-specific responses to opiates: Animal and human studies. *Anesthesia & Analgesia, 107*(1), 83–95.

D'Arcy, Y. (2009). Opioid therapy: Focus on patient safety. *American Nurse Today, 4*(5), 18–22.

Fine, P., & Portnoy, R. (2007). *A clinical guide to opioid analgesia.* New York: McGraw-Hill.

Janicki, P. K., Schuler, G., Francis, D., Bohr, A., Gordin, V., Jarzembowski, T., . . . Mets, B. (2006). A genetic association study of the functional A118G polymorphism of the human mu-opioid receptor gene in patients with acute and chronic pain. *Anesthesia & Analgesia, 103*(4), 1011–1017.

Indelicato, R. A., & Portnoy, R. K. (2002). Opioid rotation in the management of refractory cancer pain. *Journal of Clinical Oncology, 20*(1), 348–352.

Inturrisi, C., & Lipman, A. (2010). Opioid analgesics. In S. M. Fishman, J. C. Ballantyne, & J. P. Rathmell (Eds.), *Bonica's management of pain* (pp. 1174–1175). Baltimore, MD: Lippincott Williams & Wilkins.

Landau, R. (2006). One size does note fit all: Genetic variability of mu-opioid receptor and postoperative morphine consumption. *Anesthesiology, 105*(2), 235–237.

Mogil, J. (2006). Interactions between sex and genotype in mediation and modulation of nociception in rodents. In *Sex, Gender and Pain*. IASP Press: Seattle WA. pp. 25–41.

Pasternak, G. W. (2005). Molecular biology of opioid analgesia. *Journal of Pain and Symptom Management, 29*(Suppl. 5), S2–S9.

Quigley, C. (2004). Opioid switching to improve pain relief and drug tolerability. *The Cochrane Database of Systemic Reviews* (3), CD004847.

Rowbotham, M., Kidd, B., & Porecca, F. (2006). *Role of central sensitization in chronic pain: Osteoarthritis and rheumatoid arthritis compared to neuropathy*. In H. Flor, E. Kalso, & J. Dostrovsky (Eds.). Seattle, WA: IASP Press.

Smith, H., & McCleane, G. (2009). Opioids issues. In H. Smith (Ed.), *Current therapy in pain* (pp. 408–420). Philadelphia, PA: Saunders Elsevier.

Walsh, D., Davis, M. P., Estfan, B., Legrand, S. B., Lagman, R. L., & Shaheen, P. (2004). Opioid rotation prospective longitudinal study. *Journal of Clinical Oncology, 22*(14S), 8258.

10

Complementary and Integrative Therapies for Pain Management

USING COMPLEMENTARY TECHNIQUES

Patients like to have some control over the way their pain is treated, and many of them like and are interested in using techniques that are called integrative or complementary. This does not mean that they forego standard medical care, but that they add these additional treatment options into their pain relief regimen. Patients will use hot or cold compresses, yoga, or just walking to help stay in shape and increase their ability to function. Some of the advantages of these integrative techniques include the following:

- Low or no cost
- Patients can control many of the options
- Readily available and many do not require a prescription

Many patients have a favorite, tried and true pain relief measure they use before they consider trying to find help for a pain problem. Other patients are focused on wellness and have techniques they use to relieve stress, such as yoga or relaxation, that can also be very beneficial for pain relief. Patients who have arthritis or a muscle strain or sprain will try a mild analgesic they may have in their medicine chest and a little light exercise, or heat or ice to relieve the pain. Topical creams, such as Ben Gay or Icy Hot, are very popular with older patients who have this type of pain complaint (Khatta, 2007).

Because these types of treatments are over the counter, as seen on television or promoted by word of mouth for effectiveness, there is little research to recommend one treatment option over the other. Looking for the research base in this area of medicine can be confusing to say the least, because the research may be very broad and patient outcomes may not be clearly identified. One of the best resources for information on complementary treatments is the Cochrane study group database. Available at www.cochrane.org

Because of the confusing research and outcomes information, the National Institutes of Health (NIH) is studying the use of alternative treatments and has a group called the National Center for Complementary and Alternative Medicine (NCCAM) (www.nccam.nih.gov). The goal of this group of researchers is to review all the literature support and come to some recommendations about how effective and safe these treatments are. Because there is such a big interest in using organic substances such as teas, herbal remedies, and vitamin supplements for promoting health and alleviating some forms of pain such as arthritis, this group has started a review of the herbs and supplements being used to treat common conditions. Other areas of study include energy therapies and treatments such as chiropractic manipulation and acupuncture.

The general term that refers to these methods has been shortened to complementary and alternative medicine (CAM). CAM is defined as "a group of diverse medical and health care systems, practices, and products not presently considered to be a part of conventional medicine" (American Pain Society [APS], 2006). These techniques are meant to supplement, not to replace, standard medical therapies and medication.

Most patients are a bit shy about informing their health care practitioner about extra supplements and home remedies they are using. They feel the health care provider may make them feel uncomfortable about trying something that has not been prescribed for the condition. Many patients will openly tell the health care staff about their special supplements and herbal remedies if they are asked in a nonjudgmental way. Because some of these compounds can have a drug-drug interaction with the medication, it is important for the health care provider to ask questions about these types of remedies and supplements so a full medication/supplement history is taken. Patients may not even consider this information important; however, for the health care provider, this can be an integral piece of the patient's history.

CAM techniques are attractive options for most patients. They do not require a prescription, the patient controls the use, and side effects are not common. Most medications for pain can have side effects such as constipation, sedation, or dizziness, to name a few. Cost can also be a factor. Aside from supplements and herbal remedies, there is little to no cost for relaxation, biofeedback, or imagery.

Although it is hard to find a good set of CAM therapies for acute pain, there are some that are easy to use. Hot and cold compresses and massage can be used for both acute pain in the outpatient setting and for inpatients. Aromatherapy is popular with inpatients because most hospitals have an institutional/clinical odor that can be helped with essential oils. Ginger drops on a cotton ball inserted into the pillow can provide some relief from nausea and vomiting. Lavender oil used in the same way can help calm patients. Energy therapies, such as Reiki and relaxation tapes, can provide relief and decrease stress. Some patients come into the hospital looking for and expecting to have access to CAM therapies to help with relaxation and pain relief.

Where do the patients get information about CAM therapies? Many publications, such as women's magazine and the *American Association of Retired Persons Magazine*, have articles on yoga, pool therapy, or relaxation for health and stress management. Patients are also very Internet savvy. They can search the websites for information about any therapy or supplement of interest to them. Older patients are no exception. They can find information as easily as younger patients and may be willing to try something that seems to offer a quick and easy way to relieve pain (American Geriatrics Society [AGS], 2002). Health care providers should never underestimate the power of word of mouth. Something discussed at the bridge game last evening may show up in the examining room today.

Because many Americans are open to using CAM therapies to help relieve pain, practitioners for various therapies, such as yoga or acupuncture, have become common. Patients should be encouraged to ask these practitioners about their training and expertise in the technique they are providing. There are schools for massage and certificates for practitioners of therapy such as Reiki that are given to those who have completed the classes required to practice the technique. For a patient to go to an acupuncturist with little or no training or expertise, for example, may be more harmful than helpful.

In a 1997 survey, Americans reported that they made 629 million visits to CAM practitioners (Eisenberg, 1993). In Europe and Australia, about 20% to 70% of all patients use CAM therapies (O'Hara, 2003). Primary care practitioners responded that they do not ask patients about the use of CAM therapies. Only 40% of patients volunteer information on their use of CAM therapies (O'Hara, 2003). In a 2002 survey, the NCCAM determined that the most common conditions for which patients used CAM to help relieve pain were the following:

- Back pain
- Neck pain
- Joint pain
- Arthritis
- Headache (Pierce, 2009)

There can be no doubt that many patients, both old and young, find CAM modalities helpful for pain relief.

TYPES OF COMPLEMENTARY AND ALTERNATIVE MEDICINE

Long-term pain is one of the primary reasons why patients try CAM therapies. There are some techniques however, that can also be used in acute care or a referral to a clinic practicing CAM can also be made. Many of the techniques are minimally invasive, such as acupuncture, or noninvasive, such as the energy therapies of Reiki or therapeutic touch (TT). Because many patients are attracted to this type of therapy, incorporating it into the plan of care can help track outcomes and determine benefit. Because the use of these therapeutics is controversial and research is limited, it is helpful to monitor the benefit of these therapies when they are added to a plan of care. If the patient is referred for treatment to a CAM type clinic, it is important to communicate with the CAM practitioner to ensure that the selected treatment is meeting the patient's goals of care.

Many terms are applied to CAM therapies. Terms have changed through the years and some common terms are listed hereafter. Currently, integrative is the term most often used with this category of therapeutic options.

Complementary: Techniques or additional therapies that are used in conjunction with recognized mainstream medical practices, for example, when acupuncture is used concurrently with medication for low back pain.

Alternative: This term means forgoing recognized medical therapy and using other treatments for a condition, for example, when vitamin supplements and imagery are used in place of radiation or chemotherapy for cancer treatment.

Integrative: A term coined by CAM practitioners to indicate the combined use of pharmacotherapy and nonpharmacologic methods for medical treatment. This term was first used by Dr. Andrew Weil and it is the most common term applied to CAM therapies at this time (O'Hara, 2003).

There are many different types of CAM therapies that are available for treating pain. Some are very simple to use, such as heat or cold therapy, but others require patients to be educated about using the technique, such as with biofeedback, or some require a trained practitioner to administer them, such as with TT.

The four main areas or types of CAM as defined by the NCCAM are the following:

1. **Body-based therapies**, such as heat and cold therapy, massage, and acupuncture
2. **Cognitive-behavioral approaches**, or mind-body work, such as relaxation, biofeedback, and imagery

3. **Energy medicine**, including Reiki and TT
4. **Nutritional approaches** that incorporate the use of herbs and vitamin supplements

Body-Based Therapies

Heat and Cold Therapy

Heat and cold applications are common home remedies and they are one of the most basic types of CAM therapy. Patients are comfortable with the idea of using a heating pad for back pain or applying a cold pack for a minor muscle injury. Every household has an assortment of heating pads, ice packs, and the newer versions of microwave heating pads and wraps. Most patients find more comfort in heat and prefer it over cold packs. As for research support, a Cochrane report of patients with low back pain indicates that the therapies have limited support (D'Arcy, 2007; French, Cameron, Walker, Reggars, & Esterman, 2006). However, additional information demonstrates that using a heat wrap can increase functionality in this patient population (D'Arcy, 2007; French et al, 2006).

Using a heating pad or hot pack can increase circulation to the affected area, decrease stiffness, reduce pain, and relieve muscle spasms (ASPMN, 2010; D'Arcy, 2011). When using heat, patients should be cautioned as follows:

- Use it for short periods.
- Monitor use carefully over areas of decreased circulation to avoid burns.
- Avoid placing it over areas where mentholated creams such as Ben Gay or Icy Hot have been used, which can increase the potential for skin damage.
- Heat should never be placed over a patch delivering medications such as fentanyl, medications for hypertension, or smoking cessation patches. The heat over these patches will increase the delivery of the medication to the patients and put them at risk for overdose (D'Arcy, 2010).

Ice baths, cold packs, or ice massage is helpful for decreasing the pain of sprains and strains, low back pain, and muscle spasms. Many older patients do not like the cold sensation and defer using the therapy, although it would be an effective adjunct for pain relief. The cold applications work by the following:

- Decreasing nerve conduction
- Cutaneous counterirritation
- Vasoconstriction
- Muscle relaxation
- Reduction of local and systemic metabolic activity (ASPMN, 2010)

To improve the use of heat and cold and avoid tissue damage, they should be used only for a short period. Allowing the patient to use ice as a massage can be helpful and limit application time. Patients with desensitized skin, such as those with cardiovascular disease or diabetes, should take care to monitor the application sites for skin damage. Deeper application of heat can be performed using ultrasound or diathermy. Using these techniques for deep heat applications can be helpful for spasticity, muscle spasm, edema, sprains, or contusions. Again care should be taken with areas that have tissue that does not have a normal pattern of sensitivity (ASPMN, 2010).

A common approach used by health care providers for patients with a minor ache or sprain is RICE therapy.

- **R**est
- **I**ce
- **C**ompression
- **E**levation (Berry, Covington, Dahl, Katz, & Miaskowski, 2006)

For patients with chronic pain, this technique may be less useful; however, during exacerbation of musculoskeletal pain, it may provide some added relief.

Acupuncture

Acupuncture is one of the oldest CAM therapies. It originated in China, where it was used to balance the yin and yang or energy of life forces (O'Hara, 2003). The Chinese believe that life energy forces move through chakras located in various areas of the body. If the flow of energy is blocked, weak, or in a state of imbalance, an illness or pain will occur (Khatta, 2007). Acupuncture can restore balance by opening up the chakras that are blocked and allowing the life energy to flow naturally.

Acupuncture has several different variations in practice, depending on the part of the world where the practice originates. The classic approach is Chinese, and there are medical artifacts from history that indicate that acupuncture was used as a regular part of Chinese medicine for many centuries. Acupuncture relates to the use of thin needles, and other needling techniques. For pain relief, acupuncture activates the A-delta fibers in skin and muscles, which are then conveyed to the spinal cord. It stimulates the beta endorphenergic system regulating sympathetic tone. Endorphins and other pain-blocking substances such as serotonin are released (Mamtani & Frishman, 2008).

Conditions in which acupuncture has been found to be helpful include low back pain, dental pain, and the relief of nausea associated with treatment such as chemotherapy (Mamtani & Frishman, 2008), thin needles are inserted through the skin into acupuncture points (Dillard, 2005; National Center for Complementary and Alternative Medicine [NCCAM], 2004). In some cases, once the needles are in place, they are manipulated by hand or electrically stimulated to release neurotransmitters that are helpful for pain relief (Dillard, 2005).

Conditions for which acupuncture has been used include:

- Fibromyalgia
- Osteoarthritis
- Labor pain
- Dental pain (APS, 2005; Dillard, 2005).

In a study with 570 patients with osteoarthritis receiving acupuncture, the patients in the study had improvements in function and decreased pain levels (Khatta, 2007). In a review of the therapy used for relief of low back pain, acupuncture and dry needling were found to be better than sham or no treatment for pain relief and improved function (Furlan, Brosseau, Imamura, & Irvin, 2002). For low back pain, acupuncture was found to be more effective than sham acupuncture (Chou & Huffman, 2007). In acute care, finding the right location and time frame to perform acupuncture may be the most challenging aspect.

Massage

The NIH/NCCAM defines massage as pressing, rubbing, and otherwise manipulating muscles and soft tissue in the body (NCCAM, 2004). Massage has existed in many different cultures and was perceived to be healing in nature. Massage can take several different forms, with deep tissue massage or a lighter technique. Aromatherapy can be combined with massage to make the experience more relaxing. Massage is thought to relax and lengthen muscles, allowing oxygen and increased blood flow into the affected area (NCCAM, 2004). When massage is compared with other noninvasive intervention, it produces similar effects for pain relief (Chou & Huffman, 2007). Conditions that can benefit from massage include stress, pain management, improving mobility and movement, edema, postoperative care, and preoperative settings (Calenda & Weinstein, 2008). In the US, not all insurance plans cover massage and over 90% of respondents to a survey on massage report paying for the treatment out of pocket (Calenda & Weinstein, 2008). For the purpose of pain management in a study with 500 patients, the respondents self-reported reduced pain, reduced analgesic consumption, and improved physical functioning. Since massage is basically a non-invasive technique, a trial of efficacy is warranted in the acute care setting even if the area of the body is limited to hand or foot massage.

Chiropractic

For outpatients, chiropractic treatment or adjustments, which consist of spinal manipulation and other techniques, align the body to reduce pain. The findings on using chiropractic for pain relief are mixed. For low back pain, however, there is good evidence that chiropractic therapy is effective for chronic or subacute low back pain (Chou & Huffman, 2007). When using this type of therapy it is always wise to have the patient go to an accredited therapist so that the best outcome can be expected.

Transcutaneous Electrical Nerve Stimulation (TENS)

For some acute care patients, using a TENS unit can decrease pain to more tolerable levels. To use this technique a small battery pack is attached to leads with electrodes at the end. The electrodes are placed around the painful area, sometimes adjacent to a surgical incision, and a mild current is passed over the painful area. This activates large afferent fibers that stimulate dorsal horn neurons, releasing endorphins (Sharma, 2005). Since the technique is noninvasive, if the patient feels there is no benefit to the therapy, the leads can just be removed.

Other Types of Body-Based Therapies

Other forms of body-based therapies are not well supported by research. These therapies include magnets and copper bracelets. However, those that do have support can be useful to help relieve pain.

Physical therapy for reconditioning and improving balance can help maintain the mobility and functionality of older patients (AGS, 2002; Bruckenthal & D'Arcy, 2007). A regular physical therapy program has been found to reduce pain and improve mood (Bruckenthal & D'Arcy, 2007). For low back pain, exercise has good evidence to support it for pain relief (Chou & Huffman, 2007). Yoga, a form of gently stretching exercise, has also been found effective for pain relief. Viniyoga has been found superior to regular exercise for improving functional status and the use of pain medications (Chou & Huffman, 2007). Using pool therapy, in which the patients perform the physical therapy exercises in a swimming pool, can lessen the strain on sore muscles and help support the patient's body during exercise.

Clinical Pearl

The use of cognitive behavioral therapy, progressive relaxation, exercise, interdisciplinary rehabilitation, functional restoration, and spinal manipulation have produced differences of 10 to 20 points on a 100-point visual analog scale (Chou & Huffman, 2007).

Cognitive-Behavioral Therapy

Many patients are interested in using the complementary methods of relaxation, biofeedback, self-hypnosis, and imagery to provide additional pain relief (AGS, 2002; D'Arcy, 2007). Not all patients are open to trying these techniques. For those patients who are willing to invest the time and energy in learning how to use these methods, a good outcome can be expected.

Music

For acute care patients, one simple and easy technique to use is music. It can provide a distraction and provide relaxation for a patient of any age. Music therapy is defined as the use of specific music techniques to meet physical, emotional, social, and psychologic goals and objectives (Codding & Hanser, 2008). For pain management, music has a greater effect when pain is present but as pain intensities increase the positive effect of music tends to diminish. It is thought that patients who listen to music to relieve pain are providing a competing stimulus to distract the patients from the pain they are experiencing. When using music in acute care, matching the patient's preference for music type provides the best outcome. Older patients may enjoy Benny Goodman or big band tunes while younger patients may prefer more modern songs.

Relaxation

Various types of relaxation techniques can be used to help relieve pain.

- Regulating breathing for decreased respiratory efforts;
- Relaxation tapes for progressive relaxation; and
- Relaxation exercises (D'Arcy, 2007, 2010)

Relaxation techniques have been effective for decreasing pain (Cole & Brunk, 1999). These techniques result in the reduction of physical tension, muscle relaxation, and the promotion of emotional well-being (NCCAM, 2004). Relaxation is beneficial for patients who had chronic pain or cancer pain, and for surgical patients (Dillard, 2005). For acute care patients, relaxation can be done as a one-on-one intervention by a provider trained in relaxation techniques or relaxation tapes can be provided that the patient can listen to as they feel the need. Relaxation can provide an improved sense of well-being and higher scores on quality-of-life scales (Dillard, 2005).

When patients use relaxation, they are asked to either progressively relax their muscles, starting from the top of the body and progressing to the lower extremities, or they can focus on one process, such as controlling breathing. There are prerecorded tapes with relaxation exercises on them that patients can purchase to use at certain times of the day, such as when they feel stress building or as a help for relaxing to fall asleep. The patient can keep track of progress with a pain diary or journal.

Imagery

Imagery is a form of relaxation using a mental image. When a patient uses imagery, he or she is encouraged to create a peaceful or soothing image. The patient can enjoy the feeling of comfort that the scenario provides. Images can be created by the patient or provided by tapes if the patient has difficulty developing the mental images. For example, a patient could be asked to relax and picture a beautiful beach. They are asked to smell the sea air, feel the sun on their body, and hear the sound of the surf. This image is peaceful and pleasant. The patient should choose an image that can be easily called up from memory so the technique can be used very easily when it is needed for pain relief or stress reduction.

Using imagery for pain relief can also include the use of an image that locates the area of pain, such as a headache. The patients can picture the headache as a red or dark color when pain is present. Working with the image, the patients can use relaxation and cognitive restructuring to see the headache lifting from the head, getting smaller in size, or seeing the color turning to a more peaceful and restful blue tone. This type of imagery is a little more complex, but patients can learn to use it effectively to help decrease pain.

The Arthritis Self-Management Program (ASMP) uses some mind-body techniques (AGS, 2002). These include the following:

- Education
- Cognitive restructuring
- Physical activity to reduce pain

- Problem solving
- Relaxation
- Development of communication skills to help interact with health care professionals (D'Arcy, 2010)

This program has demonstrated reduced pain that lasted more than 4 years and a cost savings of 4 to 5 times the cost of the program (Khatta, 2007)

Biofeedback, hypnosis, and meditation are other forms of relaxation techniques. Meditation or mindfulness has been found to reduce pain and help patients with chronic pain learn to cope more effectively with the condition (Khatta, 2007). If the patient can learn to quiet or center himself or herself to go through a series of images or relaxation techniques, or focus on an object, meditation can be a useful adjunct for pain control. All of the mind-body techniques discussed earlier have research support for their use and which technique works for a specific patient depends on the type of approach the patient prefers (O'Hara, 2003). Another type of therapy that may fit into this category of treatment options is animal-assisted therapy. In some cases there are just informal visits by animals such as dogs that are suited and cleared to visit patients in hospitals. In other cases the animals receive training in goal-directed therapy with a specific outcome as the end result. There are guidelines for this type of intervention developed by the Delta Society. Overall, pet therapy (no matter what type of pet) is designed to provide an outside focus, increase feelings of safety, and create a source of comfort. Given the large number of pets in the United States, most patients would welcome a visit from a pet while they are in pain or ill.

Energy Therapy

Asian cultures have used energy healing for many centuries. The idea of channeling energy from the universe through the patient to open blocked chakras is derived from the concept of Qigong, an external and internal energy life force. To use these therapies with patients in modern days, several newer energy therapies were developed, including Reiki, TT, and healing touch (Pierce, 2009).

There are some differences in the practices, but the overall concepts have a similar intent.

- The human body has an energy field that is generated from within the body to the outer world.
- There is a universal energy that flows through all living things, and it is available to them.
- Self-healing is promoted through the free-flowing energy field.
- Disease and illness may be felt in the energy field and can be felt and changed by the healing intent of the practitioner (D'Arcy, 2010; Pierce, 2009).

These energy therapies are effective for pain relief and relaxation. Two of the most commonly practiced are TT and Reiki.

Reiki

The Reiki practitioner who is performing a therapeutic session on a patient uses the natural energy of the universe and channels through the patient's body to unblock chakras or energy points. The techniques used by Reiki practitioners were developed and taught by the Buddhist monk Mikao Usui from Japan beginning in 1914 (Pierce, 2009). In basic Reiki, the Reiki practitioner places his or her hands in specific configurations on the patient's body to channel the universal energy through the chakras, opening up blocked points. In more advanced levels of practice, a Reiki practitioner transmits energy long distance to benefit a specific person (NCCAM, 2004).

Reiki has been used in Eastern cultures to ease both the mind and body. There are three levels of Reiki practice. Each level includes some additional form of energy transfer. Even with the basic level, the patient feels relaxed and experiences emotional and physical healing. The Reiki practitioner who channels the energy for the patient also receives benefit. He or she feels more relaxed and in tune with his or her own body energy after the session is completed (D'Arcy, 2010).

Studies trying to show positive benefit from Reiki have focused on patients with cancer. In a study of 24 cancer patients using Reiki or rest periods, the Reiki patients had a significant decrease in pain (Pierce, 2009).

Therapeutic Touch

Therapeutic touch was developed by two nurses who hoped it would become a part of mainstream nursing care. It is similar to Reiki but the TT practitioner does not place their hands onto the patients but holds them over the patients to do an assessment for blocked energy.

Smoothing the aura by the energy transfer from the practitioner to the patient can help provide healing energy. TT should not be mistaken for the more religious practice of the laying on of hands as a healing practice. The premise of TT is that the practitioner's healing force transfers or channels energy, thereby positively affecting the recovery of the patient (NCCAM, 2004). As the TT practitioner allows his or her hands to move over the patient, blocked energy is identified and, through the practitioner's hands, healing forces are directed to the area to promote healing and pain relief.

There are some studies that indicate greater pain relief with the use of TT in patients with chronic pain and fibromyalgia, when compared with patient groups not receiving the energy treatment option (Pierce, 2009). It is difficult to conduct a study with TT because the recipient knows that they are not receiving the actual treatment, but only a sham. Because randomized placebo-controlled studies are not possible with TT, it is difficult to measure the true effect of the practice.

Nutritional Approaches

Folk medicine and natural healing have long been a part of most cultures. Many patients feel uncomfortable sharing information on their use of supplements and herbal remedies with their health care provider. It is important to ask about these supplements and allow for an open discussion of the pros and cons of this type of therapy. Herbal remedies are some of the most common forms of complementary therapeutics (Khatta, 2007). The advantage of these therapies is that they are simple and easy to use, viewed as noninvasive, and benign with few side effects, but on the negative side, they have little or no quality control mechanism. From 1990 to 1997, herbal remedy use increased by 380% (Khatta, 2007). Cost-wise, the annual expenditure on herbal remedies in the United States exceeded $1.5 billion (Khatta, 2007).

Many of the early tonics and elixirs peddled in early American towns and settlements had cocaine or high alcohol contents with flavorings to make them palatable. Laudanum was a popular elixir used for pain relief, from childbirth to war injuries. Today, all dietary supplements are categorized under the Dietary Supplement Health and Education Act of 1994, which requires quality, safety, and efficacy standards. However, there are still discrepancies in contents of some of the supplements and herbal remedies sold over the counter, so, as always, the buyer should be wary of what they are purchasing. This is especially true for pregnant and compromised patients. Common herbal remedies include the following:

- Cayenne (Capsicum). Cayenne can be made into plasters and placed over the painful areas. Capsaicin is the active ingredient of cayenne peppers (Khatta, 2007). Capsaicin is sold as an over-the-counter cream as a generic product or with brand name (Zostrix). The cream produces a strong sensation of heat, and it can also burn and sting. It comes in two strengths and should be carefully applied while the patient is wearing gloves to protect the areas that are not painful. Patients who are using capsaicin should apply the cream 3 to 4 times daily over at least 2 weeks to see any improvement. When applying capsaicin cream, wearing gloves is advised and care with touching other parts of the body, especially the eyes, is recommended. A new 8% topical Capsaicin patch has been developed (Quetensa) for topical application in herpes zoster patients who develop postherpetic neuralgia (PHN), a very painful condition. This patch needs to have a local anesthetic applied over the application area prior to patch placement. The patch must be placed by a medical professional and removed in exactly one hour. The benefit is a good level of pain relief that can last for up to 12 weeks.
- Devil's claw (*Harpagophytum procumbens*). Use of this herb in patients with osteoarthritis resulted in a reduction in pain levels and an increase in mobility (Khatta, 2007).

- Willow bark (*Salix alba*). The results for this herb are inconsistent, and only short-term improvement has been demonstrated (Khatta, 2007).
- One frequently used herb, *Corydalis*, is an alkaloid with potent analgesic properties (Dillard, 2005). It traditionally has been used for menstrual pain.

Nutritional supplements include the following:

- One of the most popular and disputed supplements for arthritis pain is glucosamine and chondroitin. Studies have shown a slowing of disease progression over time and that combination medications can affect pain in osteoarthritis patients (Khatta, 2007).
- Omega-3 fatty acids affect prostaglandin metabolism, thereby affecting the inflammatory process. Fish oil has been found to have anti-inflammatory effects in patients with rheumatoid arthritis, whereas flaxseed oil has no similar effect (Khatta, 2007).

Patients who are taking nutritional supplements and herbal remedies should tell their primary care provider that they are using the substances. Although there is the potential for drug-drug interactions with mainstream medications, every patient should be asked if they are taking a supplement or herbal remedy. Only those supplements and herbs that have shown efficacy in clinical trials and are recommended by the NCCAM should be used for complementary pain relief.

SUMMARY

Acute care can be a difficult place to use complementary therapies. Outpatient settings offer much more opportunity for a trial of these therapies. Trying the techniques one at a time and choosing one that the patient feels may be effective is a way to introduce the patient to the idea of using a different approach to pain control. Once the patient is comfortable with a new idea about pain control, they may be more open to trying a variety of techniques that will in the end provide a better outcome than medication alone.

Case Study

Your neighbor Susanne tells you she has hurt her back recently while moving some heavy furniture in her house. She says the pain is about a 6/10 and it stays there all the time. Her doctor told her there was nothing wrong with her back and it would be better in time. She can barely bring herself to get out of bed in the morning. She is stiff and her muscles just seem to be tight in her lower back. She tries to stay up on her feet, but the pain has gotten to be such a problem for her, and it does not seem to get any better. She has been taking acetaminophen for the pain, and she wonders if there is some kind of home remedy or nonpharmacologic technique that would help her. She hates pain medicine and gets sick every time she takes it. What would you suggest for her pain?

Questions to Consider

1. Because Susanne has been seen by her doctor who has not found any cause for her pain, what types of CAM therapies could be used?
2. Would Susanne be a candidate for acupuncture, TENS, or chiropractic manipulation?
3. After Susanne finds a way to decrease her pain, what types of mind-body or cognitive-behavioral techniques could she use?
4. Would any of the topical agents or supplements help Susanne's pain?
5. After Susanne's pain improves, would a regular yoga class help maintain her muscle strength and flexibility?

REFERENCES

American Geriatrics Society. (2002). The management of persistent pain in older persons. *Journal of the American Geriatrics Society, 50*(Suppl. 6), S205–S224.

American Pain Society. (2002). *Guideline for the management of pain in osteoarthritis, rheumatoid arthritis, and juvenile chronic arthritis.* Glenview, IL: Author.

American Pain Society. (2005). *Guideline for the management of fibromyalgia syndrome pain in adults and children.* Glenview, IL: Author.

American Pain Society. (2006). *Pain control in the primary care setting.* Glenview, IL: Author.

American Society of Pain Management Nursing. (2010). *Core curriculum for pain management nursing.* Dubuque, IA: Kendall Hunt Publishing.

Berry, P., Covington, E., Dahl, J., Katz, J., & Miaskowski, C. (2006). *Pain: Current understanding of assessment, management, and treatments.* Reston, VA: National Pharmaceutical Council, Inc.

Bruckenthal, P., & D'Arcy, Y. (2007). A complementary approach to pain management. *Topics in Advanced Practice Nursing eJournal, 7*(1). Retrieved from http://www.medscape.com/viewarticle/556408

Calenda, E., & Weinstein, S. (2008). *Therapeutic massage in complementary and integrative medicine in pain management.* New York, NY: Springer.

Chou, R., & Huffman, L. (2007). Nonpharmacologic therapies for acute and chronic low back pain: A review of the evidence for an American Pain Society/American College of Physicians clinical practice guideline. *Annals of Internal Medicine, 147*(7), 492–504.

Codding, P., & Hanser, S. (2008). *Music therapy in complementary and integrative medicine in pain management.* New York, NY: Springer Publishing.

Cole, B. H., & Brunk, Q. (1999). Holistic interventions for acute pain episodes: An integrative review. *Journal of Holistic Nursing, 17*(4), 384–396.

D'Arcy, Y. (2007). *Pain management: Evidence-based tools and techniques for nursing professionals.* Marblehead, MA: HCPro.

D'Arcy, Y. (2010). *How to treat pain in the elderly.* Indianapolis, IN: Sigma Theta Tau.

D'Arcy, Y. (2011). *Compact clinical guide to chronic pain management: An evidence-based approach for nurses.* New York, NY: Springer Publishing.

Dillard, J. N., & Knapp, S. (2005). Complementary and alternative pain therapy in the emergency department. *Emergency Medical Clinics of North America, 23*(2), 529–549.

Eisenberg, D. M., Kessler, R. C., Foster, C., Norlock, F. E., Calkins, D. R., & Delbanco, T. L. (1993). Unconventional medicine in the United States: Prevalence, costs, and patterns of use. *New England Journal of Medicine, 328*(4), 246–252.

French, S. D., Cameron, M., Walker, B. F., Reggars, J. W., & Esterman, A. J. (2006). Superficial heat or cold for low back pain. *Cochrane Database of Systemic Reviews* (1).

Furlan, A. D., Brosseau, L., Imamura, M., & Irvin, E. (2006). Massage for low back pain. *Cochrane Database of Systematic Reviews* (2).

Khatta, M. (2007). A complementary approach to pain management. *Topics in Advanced Practice Nursing eJournal,* 7(1). Retrieved from http://www.medscape.com/viewarticle/556408

Mamtani, R., & Frishman, W. (2008). *Acupuncture in complementary and integrative medicine in pain management.* New York, NY: Springer.

National Center for Complementary and Alternative Medicine. (2004). *Expanding Horizons of Health Care Strategic Plan 2005–2009.* Bethesda, MD: U.S. Department of Health and Human Services. National Institutes of Health. Retrieved from www.nccam.nih.gov

O'Hara, D. A. (2003). Pain management. In P. Iyer (Ed.), *Medical–legal aspects of suffering*. Tucson, AZ: Lawyers and Judges Publishing.

Pierce, B. (2009). A nonpharmacologic adjunct for pain management. *The Nurse Practitioner, 34*(2), 10–13.

Sharma, M. (2005). Complementary and alternative medicine. In M. Wallace & M. Staats (Eds.), *Pain medicine & management: Just the facts* (pp. 227–282). New York, NY: McGraw-Hill.

IV

Advanced Pain Management Techniques

11

Perioperative Pain Management

Acute pain is the natural result of surgery, a procedure, or injury. Patients expect acute pain to resolve once the recovery period is complete. For the surgical patient, pain management begins before surgery and continues through discharge; the perioperative period consists of the preoperative, intraoperative, and postoperative periods. Each area plays a very important role in the success of pain management. The quality of pain relief provided during the perioperative period can impact the type of recovery either positively or negatively and can affect long-term outcomes.

In a study of 342 patients undergoing surgery, postoperative morphine use was tracked to determine predictive factors for postoperative pain. The findings indicate that those patients, who had higher doses of intraoperative sufentanil, general anesthesia, or preoperative treatment with analgesics and preoperative benzodiazepines, all had a much higher potential for severe postoperative pain (Aubrun, Valade, Coriat, & Riou, 2008). Predictive factors for morphine consumption in the postoperative period were identified as emergency surgery, a surgical procedure lasting longer than 100 minutes, a pain score of 2 or 3 on a scale of 5 on arrival to the postanesthesia care unit (PACU) (Ip, Abrishami, Peng, Wong, & Chung, 2009), Caucasian patients, and major surgery (Aubrun et al., 2008). Knowing which patient might have a need for more aggressive pain management in the postoperative period can help stratify care for patients who are being sent to the PACU.

The length of time that pain can be moderate to severe after surgery depends on the type of surgical procedure and the type of pain relief provided during the perioperative period. The mean number of days for moderate to severe postoperative pain ranges from 8 days for intrathoracic surgery to 1 day for both appendectomy and head and neck surgery (Palomano, Rathmell, Krenzischek, & Dunwoody, 2008). Because best estimates indicate that 73 million surgeries are performed annually, with 80% of the patients experiencing pain after surgery and with 86% of these patient groups reporting moderate to severe pain (Apfelbaum, Chen, Mehta, & Gan, 2003), perioperative pain management is an important aspect of acute pain management.

With the advances in science, pharmacology, and medical practice, pain management can start before surgery and continue throughout the perioperative period. For operative and postoperative pain relief, anesthesiologists have developed new techniques for combining different types of pain management, including opioids, local anesthetic infusions, and neuraxial blocks. The idea that perioperative pain has been undermanaged in all surgical areas is not a new concept but it has been difficult to capture data. Postoperative pain continues to be one of the most commonly reported symptoms (Apfelbaum et al., 2003). If the pain is untreated or undertreated, persistent acute pain can have several negative effects. Patients may have negative perceptions of postoperative pain management and fear unrelieved pain after their surgery. Depending on the level of anxiety about postoperative pain management, pain levels can be increased if anxiety levels are high.

Acute pain can progress into a more difficult-to-treat chronic pain syndrome, such as a naturopathic pain syndrome, complex regional pain syndrome, or postthoracotomy pain syndrome (American Pain Society [APS], 2008; Macrae, 2001; Palomano et al., 2008; Perkins & Kehlet, 2000). If the acute pain is not treated adequately, it can have negative effects on the patient's body as healing tries to occur, such as adverse effects on the immune and endocrine systems (Page, 2005), that also lead to effects on cardiopulmonary and thromboembolic diseases (Ballatyne et al., 1998; Beattie, Buckley, & Forrest, 1993). Myocardial ischemia and infarction may be caused by reduced myocardial oxygen supply and increased myocardial oxygen consumption (Liu et al., 1995; Wu & Fleisher, 2000). The additive effects can also cause a delay in wound healing (Akca et al., 1999).

In addition to the physiologic effects of inadequately treated acute perioperative pain, the increased emotional and physiologic distress can add to the pain and decrease the effectiveness of the treatments being used to relieve the pain. About 59% of all patients who are having surgery report that postoperative pain management is a concern for them (Apfelbaum et al., 2003). If pain relief is ineffective, this lack of pain relief can create a significant morbidity for the patient that can affect recovery (Hurley, Cohen, & Wu, 2010).

Clinical Pearl

Unrelieved perioperative pain can have negative consequences that include physiologic effects, such as negative effect on the immune and endocrine systems, increased potential for cardiac ischemia, delayed wound healing, emotional distress, impaired coping, and lack of progression toward recovery with delayed discharge.

BEFORE SURGERY

If the patient is being seen by his or her own health care provider prior to a planned surgery, the records of all medications and chronic conditions will be in the office records, and the information should be given to the hospital where the surgery is planned. A current history and physical (H&P) is usually required within 30 days of the anticipated surgery. Some hospitals offer a presurgical service that induces the H&P and all needed referrals and laboratory work. Whichever way the patient reaches the operating room, the H&P must be up to date and reflect all medical conditions, current laboratory values, and medications that could affect surgery.

For many patients, the preholding area is the first contact the patient will have with the hospital staff. Information gathered in the preholding area is vital to the success of the surgery and postoperative pain management. The patient may be anxious about the upcoming surgery and need reassurance. The information gathered in this area, especially a pain management history, can provide important information about past experiences with pain management and pain medication usage and allergies to specific opioid medications.

Information that should be gathered in the preholding area related to past pain management includes the following:

- Vital signs
- A pain assessment using a tool such as the 0 to 10 Numeric Rating Scale (NRS), FACES for children, or Pain Assessment in Advanced Dementia (PAINAD) for demented patients
- Medical history—looking for chronic pain conditions, such as fibromyalgia or rheumatoid arthritis, that can affect postoperative pain relief
- Pain history—if the patient has had difficulty with pain management in the past, what medications do and do not work for pain relief, and any issues surrounding past pain management, such as nausea and vomiting with specific pain medications
- Patient preferences—what type of pain management is hoped to be received by the patient
- Current medication history—what types of pain medication the patient has been taking regularly, what dose, and how long the patient has been taking these medications
- Substance use history, alcohol use, illicit substances, or tobacco use.

Patients on opioid therapy should take their usual morning medications to avoid an abstinence syndrome or lack of treatment of preexisting pain (ASA, 2004).

It is crucial for the medical staff in the preholding area to get an accurate count of what opioids are being used currently, as well as their correct doses. If the patient does not have this information, the primary health care provider or pain management specialist who orders these medications should be contacted to ensure that the patient has the correct drug and doses to avoid undertreating or overdosing after surgery. Some patients with chronic pain may fear unrelieved pain after surgery and report higher doses of current pain medications in order to make sure they have adequate medication in the postoperative time period. It is crucial to obtain the actual dose of opioid that the patient is currently taking at the time of surgery so that the patient does not become oversedated. If time permits, educating the patient about patient-controlled analgesia (PCA), telling the patient that it is important to report pain, and reviewing how to report pain after surgery are helpful for the patient when he or she gets to the postoperative unit. Unfortunately, many patients have high anxiety prior to surgery, and education may not be well absorbed by the patient in the preoperative area.

Preemptive Analgesia

Preemptive analgesia is the use of a medication or a technique such as surgical site infiltration with local anesthetic prior to surgery in hopes of reducing postoperative pain. The concept is controversial and findings are mixed. A systematic review by Katz and McCartney (2002) found no benefit with preemptive strategies. In a review of preemptive studies, D'Arcy (2008) found that the techniques and surgical procedures that had no benefit from preemptive analgesia were oral medications, including opioids and nonsteroidal anti-inflammatory drugs (NSAIDs), surgical site infiltration with local anesthethic, intravenous (IV) pain medication, and epidural analgesia placed during surgery. The only procedure that had any benefit from preemptive analgesia was breast surgery. In all the studies included for review, pain scores, which are the most important factor postoperatively, were not reduced by any of the forms of preemptive analgesia, and many were remarkably similar to the patients who did not receive any preemptive intervention (D'Arcy, 2008).

Looking beyond opioids and local anesthetic infiltration, a systematic review of 22 studies found that a single dose of gabapentin ranging from 300 to 1,200 mg given 1 to 2 hours preoperatively improved pain relief; reduced opioid usage by 20% to 62%; and prevented and reduced opioid side effects, such as nausea, vomiting, and urinary retention. Sedation was the most common side effect with the gabapentin group (Tippana, Hamunen, Kontinen, & Kalso, 2007).

The concept of preemptive analgesia is a good idea because reducing pain before it can fully activate and gets severe is an attractive goal. Although preemptive analgesia seems to be a good option, most studies seem to indicate that there is little or no benefit from preemptive analgesia in most cases, gabapentinoids such as gabapentin (Neurontin) and pregabalin (Lyrica) being the exception.

INTRAOPERATIVE PAIN MANAGEMENT

Pain stimuli are being sent to the patient who is under anesthesia that can result in a central sensitization phenomenon as a result of continued pain transmission from the periphery (Pogatzki-Zahn & Zahn, 2006). Because of this continued input of pain stimuli, it is important that pain control continues in the intraoperative period, even though the patient is sedated and unable to report pain.

Current recommendations include the use of multimodal therapies to help control pain during the intraoperative period and into the postoperative period (Hurley, Cohen, & Wu, 2010). Epidural or intrathecal opioids; neuraxial blocks, such as interpleural, plexus, intercostal, ilioinguinal, or penile blocks; and systemic opioids may be combined to have good effects. Commonly used opioids in the operating room include fentanyl (Sublimaze), sufentanil (Sufenta), morphine, or hydromorphone (Dilaudid) (ASA, 2004). Because some of the opioids can cause adverse effects, many times patients are given an antiemetic to counteract the overall effects of medications used during the intraoperative period. Patients who have pain management techniques implemented during surgery, such as intraoperative blocks, reach the postoperative area with a higher level of pain control after surgery.

POSTOPERATIVE PAIN MANAGEMENT

The choices for postoperative pain management include opioids administered either by epidural, PCA, or intravenously; multimodal therapies, including blocks; and other medications, such as acetaminophen, NSAIDs, anticonvulsants, or gabapentinoid medications.

The epidural route provides the largest amount of pain relief with the lowest dose of medication; however, not all surgical cases are candidates for epidural pain management. Patients who are good candidates for epidural pain management include those who had large abdominal surgeries, thoracotomies, and joint replacements. Recommended medications for use in postoperative epidural catheters include morphine and fentanyl, with hydromorphone and sufentanil having less evidence for use. Although there is a high rate of pruritus and urinary retention with morphine, when given via epidural, the pain relief is superior to either IV or intramuscular morphine (ASA, 2004). More information on epidural pain management will be provided in Chapter 13.

Another commonly used option for pain relief in the postoperative period is IV opioids, given either as intermittent doses administered by nurses as needed or as a PCA that patients can use as needed. The obvious drawback to intermittent IV doses of medication is the time delay from the patient feeling the pain to the nurse being able to provide the medication. To eliminate the delay factor, a PCA can be used when the patient is able to self-deliver a dose of opioid medication when the pain starts. Common medications prescribed for PCA use include morphine, hydromorphone (Dilaudid), and fentanyl (Sublimaze). The use of opioids for postoperative pain control can cause adverse effects, such as nausea, pruritus, constipation, and urinary retention. It is important that patients who are taking opioids regularly for postoperative pain relief be given laxatives to maintain regular bowel function. More information on PCA use will be provided in Chapter 12.

Clinical Pearl

The use of a standard order set in the PACU area can give guidance and offer options for both pain control and postoperative nausea and vomiting. See PACU order set in Figure 11.1.

The multimodal approach to postoperative pain relief may also include the use of a peripheral nerve catheter or a catheter threaded along an incision providing local anesthetic to reduce pain. These techniques are recommended especially for certain surgeries, such as

ANESTHESIA ORDERS

POST ANESTHESIA CARE UNIT
STANDING ORDERS

ALLERGIES ➤

PATIENT PLATE

Admit to PACU. Discharge from PACU when criteria met.

☐ Fast Track

Oxygen via: NC _____ liters / min FM/Face Tent ____ % Non-rebreather mask ____ %

Ventilatory settings: Tidal Volume _____ Mode _____ Rate _____ FiO2 _____ Peep _____

IV Fluid: ____________ @ _______ cc / h

☐ Fingerstick (call if > ____ or < ____) ☐ ISTAT ☐ PCXR ☐ ABGs ☐ 12 Lead EKG

Patient parameters and medical condition / history must be considered prior to administration of any medications ordered

DO NOT ADMINISTER NARCOTICS IF RESPIRATORY RATE IS < 10 / MINUTE, SEDATION SCALE is > 2, or patient states pain level is tolerable.

☐ **Morphine Sulfate:** dose to be administered every ☐ 5 minutes **or** every ☐ 10 minutes PRN pain
- 2 mg IV of Morphine Sulfate for mild pain (1 – 3 /10)
- 3 mg IV of Morphine Sulfate for moderate pain (4 – 6 /10)
- 4 mg IV of Morphine Sulfate for severe pain (7 – 10 /10)
- Notify anesthesiologist when total dose reaches _____ and pain remains > 4 /10

☐ **Fentanyl:** dose to be administered every ☐ 5 minutes **or** every ☐ 10 minutes PRN pain
- 12.5 micrograms IV of Fentanyl for mild pain (1 – 3 /10)
- 25 micrograms IV of Fentanyl for moderate pain (4 – 6 /10)
- 50 micrograms IV of Fentanyl for severe pain (7 – 10 /10)
- Notify anesthesiologist when total dose reaches _____ and pain remains > 4 /10

☐ **Hydromorphone:** dose to be administered every ☐ 5 minutes **or** every ☐ 10 minutes PRN pain
- 0.2 mg IV of Hydromorphone for mild pain (1 – 3 /10)
- 0.3 mg IV of Hydromorphone for moderate pain (4 – 6 /10)
- 0.5 mg IV of Hydromorphone for severe pain (7 – 10 /10)
- Notify anesthesiologist when total dose reaches _____ and pain remains > 4 /10

☐ Hydrocodone and Acetaminophen (5 mg / 500 mg) _____ tab(s) po x 1 in PACU PRN pain
☐ Oxycodone and Acetaminophen (5 mg / 325 mg) _____ tab(s) po x 1 in PACU PRN pain
☐ Hydromorphone _____ mg po x 1 in PACU PRN pain

Nausea and Vomiting

☐ Ondansetron 2 mg IV; may repeat x 1 in _____ minutes
☐ Promethazine _____ mg IV PRN x 1; may repeat x 1 in _____ minutes
☐ Metoclopramide 10 mg IV; may repeat x 1 in _____ minutes

Additional PACU orders:

☐ Ketorolac _____ mg IVP x 1 for pain
☐ Meperidine _____ mg IV every _____ min. in PACU PRN shivering
☐ Labetalol _____ mg IV every 5 minutes PRN systolic BP > _____ or diastolic BP > _____
☐ Hydralazine _____ mg IV every _____ minutes PRN systolic BP > _____ or diastolic BP > _____

RN SIGNATURE	PHYSICIAN SIGNATURE	DATE	TIME

PATIENT SAFETY ALERT

USE	Do not use
DAILY	QD
EVERY OTHER DAY	QOD
UNITS	U
0.5 MG.	Lack of leading zero (e.g. .5 mg)
10 MG.	Trailing zero (e.g. 10.0 mg)
MORPHINE SULFATE	MS or MSO4
MAGNESIUM SULFATE	MgSO4
MICRO-GRAM OR MCG.	µg or µ for microgram
INTER-NATIONAL UNITS	IU
LEFT EAR; RIGHT EAR; BOTH EARS	A.S.; A.D.; A.U.
LEFT EYE; RIGHT EYE; BOTH EYES;	O.S.; O.D.; O.U.

Figure 11.1 ■ Order set exemplar. *Source:* Courtesy of Suburban Hospital–Johns Hopkins Medicine, Bethesda, MD.

orthopedic joint replacement, and surgeries with large incisions, such as open nephrectomies.

As the patient progresses in recovery, oral medication can be substituted for the IV medications, and the patient can be tapered off of the medications as the pain resolves. Patients who continue to complain of high levels of unrelieved pain in the postoperative period should be assessed for a neuropathic source for their pain that would require a different type of medication for pain management.

THE USE OF GUIDELINES AND STANDARDS FOR ACUTE PAIN MANAGEMENT

There are various pain management standards and guidelines for use in the acute care postoperative setting. These guidelines can provide a base for ensuring that every patient has his or her pain assessed and treated. Each hospital and surgical center has policies and guidelines that govern how a patient who had surgery has their pain assessed and receives pain control. In addition to these formal written tools, the hospital or facility needs to monitor compliance with these policies to ensure that health care providers and staff are compliant with the recommendations.

For hospitals, The Joint Commission monitors pain management practice. Some techniques, such as hospital-wide pain management protocols, have either proved effective or increased postoperative sedation (D'Arcy & Johann, 2008; Nevius & D'Arcy, 2009; Vila et al., 2005). Whatever method, technique, or combination of modalities is used for perioperative pain relief, the patient who receives adequate pain assessment and management will progress to discharge sooner and with less physiologic strain.

For ambulatory care surgical centers, it is important to maximize pain control in the postoperative period and aggressively control adverse side effects, such as nausea, vomiting, and sedation. Because 70% of all surgeries have moved to ambulatory care centers (Apfelbaum et al., 2003), the need for effective pain relief with few, if any, side effects has increased. Perioperative pain management in both inpatient and outpatient settings is more critical than it was in the past, with more emphasis being placed on using pain management to progress the patient to a timely discharge.

Case Study

Peter Jones, a 17-year-old trauma patient, is admitted to the emergency department (ED) after a high-speed traffic accident. The officers at the scene report that the vehicle Peter was driving hit another vehicle and was forced into the guardrail. Peter's injuries include a fractured left femur, multiple rib fractures, and a large open wound along the anterior aspect of his left leg. He also has a concussion. He is assessed as able to tolerate surgery. Before he is transported to surgery, he spends 3 hours in the ED and is given several doses of morphine IV after a urine screen has been sent to the laboratory. He continues to complain of severe level pain right up to the time of surgery.

When Peter comes out of surgery, he is moaning and complaining of severe level pain. The PACU nurses keep administering doses of IV morphine, but nothing seems to touch Peter's pain. Peter is given a hydromorphone PCA but he still has unrelieved pain. When Peter's urine screen is returned, it shows that he is positive for marijuana, opiates, and benzodiazepines. What can be done to make Peter's pain relief better?

Questions to Consider

1. Does Peter's age make a difference in his ability to understand his pain and allow him to have realistic expectations?
2. Does his substance abuse play a part in his unrelieved pain? Would higher medication doses resolve his lack of pain relief?
3. What combination of medications and techniques would work best for Peter's pain management?
4. Would doses of medication in the operating room have helped Peter? Do you think the source of his unrelieved pain is not achieving an adequate blood level of medication before being placed on the PCA?
5. Does his concussion preclude the use of opioids?

REFERENCES

Akca, O., Melischek, M., Scheck, T., Hellwagner, K., Arklas, C. F., Kurtz, A., . . . Sessler, D. I. (1999). Postoperative pain and subcutaneous oxygen tension. *Lancet*, *354*(9172), 41–42.

American Pain Society. (2008). *Principles of analgesic use in the treatment of acute pain and cancer pain*. Glenview, IL: Author.

American Society of Anesthesiologists Task Force on Acute Pain Management. (2004). Practice guidelines for acute pain management in the perioperative setting. *Anesthesiology*, *100*(6), 1573–1581.

Apfelbaum, J. L., Chen, C., Mehta, S. S., & Gan, T. J. (2003). Postoperative pain experience: Results from a national survey suggest postoperative pain continues to be undermanaged. *Anesthesia & Analgesia*, *97*(2), 534–540.

Aubrun, F., Valade, N., Coriat, P., & Riou, B. (2008). Predictive factors of severe postoperative pain in the post anesthesia care unit. *Anesthesia & Analgesia*, *106*(5), 1535–1541.

Ballantyne, B., Carr, D., DeForantin, S., Suarez, T., Lau, J., Chalmers, T. C., . . . Mosteller, F. (1998). The comparative effects of postoperative analgesic therapies on pulmonary outcome: A cumulative meta-analysis of randomized, controlled trials. *Anesthesia and Analgesia*, *86*(3), 598–612.

Beattie, W. S., Buckley, D. N., & Forrest, J. B. (1993). Epidural morphine reduces the risk of postoperative myocardial ischemia in patients with cardiac risk factors. *Canadian Journal of Anesthesia*, *40*(6), 532–541.

D'Arcy, Y. (2008). First strike: Does preemptive analgesia work? *Nursing, 38*(4), 52–55.

D'Arcy, Y., & Johann, D. (2008). Using a medication protocol to improve pain management. *Nursing Management, 39*(3), 35–39.

Hurley, W., Cohen, S., & Wu, C. (2010). Acute pain in adults. In *Bonica's management of pain* (pp. 699–751). Philadelphia, PA: Lippincott Williams & Wilkins.

Ip, H. Y., Abrishami, A., Peng, P. W., Wong, J., & Chung, F. (2009). Predictors of postoperative pain and analgesic consumption. *Anesthesiology, 111*, 657–677.

Katz, J., & McCartney, C. J. (2002). Current status of preemptive analgesia. *Current Opinion in Anaesthesiology, 15*, 435–441.

Liu, S., Carpenter, R. L., Mulroy, M. F., Weissman, R. M., McGill, T. J., Rupp, S. M., & Allen, H. W. (1995). Intravenous versus epidural administration of hydromorphone. Effects on analgesia and recovery after radical retropubic prostatectomy. *Anesthesiology, 82*(3), 682–688.

Macrae, W. A. (2001). Chronic pain after surgery. *British Journal of Anaesthesia, 87*(1), 88–98.

Nevius, K., & D'Arcy, Y. (2009). Decrease recovery time with proper pain management. *Nursing Management, 39*(1), 26–32.

Page, G. (2005). Surgery-induced immunosuppression and postoperative pain management. *ACCN Clinical Issues, 16*(3), 302–309.

Palomano, R. C., Rathmell, J. P., Krenzischek, D. A., & Dunwoody, C. J. (2008). Emerging trends and new approaches to acute pain management. *Pain Management Nursing, 9*(1), S33–S41.

Perkins, F. M., & Kehlet, H. (2000). Chronic pain as an outcome of surgery: A review of predictive factors. *Anesthesiology, 93*(4), 1123–1133.

Pogatzki-Zahn, E. M., & Zahn, P. K. (2006). From preemptive to preventive analgesia. *Current Opinions in Anaesthesiology, 19*, 551–555.

Tippana, E. M., Hamunen, K., Kontinen, V. K., & Kalso, E. (2007). Do surgical patients benefit from perioperative gabapentin/pregabalin? A systematic review of efficacy and safety. *Anesthesia & Analgesia, 104*(6), 1545–1556.

Vila, H., Smith, R., Augustyniak, M., Nagi, P., Soto, R., Ross, T., . . . Miguel, R. (2005). The efficacy and safety of pain management before and after implementation of hospital-wide pain management standards: Is patient safety compromised by treatment based solely on numerical pain ratings? *Anesthesia & Analgesia, 101*(2), 474–480.

Wu, C. L., & Fleisher, L. A. (2000). Outcomes research in regional anesthesia and analgesia. *Anesthesia & Analgesia, 91*(5), 1232–1242.

12

Patient-Controlled Analgesia

OVERVIEW OF PCA

Patient-controlled analgesia (PCA) is more than the machine used to deliver the medication; it is a process. This process consists of the patient, the delivery system, and the medications with dosing parameters. If any one of these elements is eliminated, the process should no longer be considered PCA.

The PCA system consists of a computerized pump that delivers opioid medication through intravenous (IV) tubing into the patient's IV access. The patient is able to activate the machine using a push-button device when pain increases. Once the button is pushed, the pump delivers a preset dose of medication to the patient. The pump is programmed by the nursing staff according to PCA orders written by a licensed prescriber. The pump can be set to deliver several different types of prefilled opioid syringes, cassettes, or bags and can be programmed to deliver a continuous or basal dose along with a patient-activated bolus dose.

Most patients prefer PCA to other forms of postoperative analgesia because they have some control over their pain relief. They can use the medication when they feel pain and do not have to wait for the nurse to answer a call light, get the medication from a medication machine (Pyxis), and then return to the patient's room to deliver the medication. The ease of PCA and quick response time for medication delivery are very attractive for patients. A Cochrane review of 55 studies with 2,023 patients reported that PCA provided better pain relief and increased patient satisfaction compared with as-needed (PRN) medication dosing, but the patients also had a higher medication use and increased pruritis compared with patients using standard means of postoperative pain management (Hudcova, McNicol, Quah, Lau, & Carr, 2006).

The first PCAs were developed in the 1970s in an effort to improve on the standard forms of postoperative pain control (i.e., intermittent intramuscular [IM] injections of opioids provided by a nurse). The older forms of medication administration allowed for a period of oversedation, then a period of pain relief, followed by a period of pain or end-of-dose failure as the medication dissipated. Because of the potential for irregular medication absorption, IM injections are no longer recommended for pain management (American Pain Society [APS], 2008). Blood levels of medication fluctuate and exceed the patient's needs and then, as blood levels decrease, the patient experiences pain. Very often, as pain returns, the patient would be told that "It is not time for your medication," and the patient would be forced to wait in pain until the stipulated time was reached. Studies conducted on PCA in the early 1970s indicated that small doses of medication given at regular intervals provided superior pain relief to the standard IM injections, and it eliminated the variation in pain relief with intermittent injections (Grass, 2005).

Each patient has an individual blood level of medication that will provide analgesia. With PCA, the patient should be medicated with IV loading doses until an acceptable level of pain relief is achieved, allowing the patient to maintain pain control with bolus doses. With PCA machines, no matter how often patients push the button, they will receive only the dose that is programmed into the pump in the preset lockout time. If a patient starts to become sedated, he or she will stop pushing the button. If the patient falls asleep, he or she will usually wake and use the button as pain returns.

PATIENT-CONTROLLED ANALGESIA MEDICATIONS AND ORDERS

There are several medications and medication combinations that can be used in PCA pumps (see Table 12.1). The most common opioids are morphine, hydromorphone (Dilaudid), and fentanyl (Sublimaze). Other medications, such as methadone (Dolophine) and buprenorphine (Buprenex), can also be used but have more specific actions, such as extended half-life for methadone and mixed agonist–antagonist activity for buprenorphine (Buprenex), and these medications are used for specific indications, such as rare instances of methadone for highly opioid-dependent patients with cancer pain. Each medication has a benefit that can be used to maximize pain relief for a patient. Each patient also has a genetic uniqueness that makes some types of medication work most effectively. Pairing the right medication with the patient's genetic predisposition and metabolism characteristics can provide the best pain relief possible. Looking at how effective pain relief is with a specific medication can indicate that the patient's genetic makeup accepts the medication effectively for pain relief without having to genetically profile the patient.

Clinical Pearl

The binding ability and activity of a medication being used for PCA are, in part, related to its chemical structure. For example, morphine is hydrophilic (water loving) and tends to spread throughout the body in the aqueous regions. Because the spread is so wide, it tends to remain active for a longer period. Fentanyl, on the other hand, is lipophilic (fat loving), crosses the blood-brain barrier easily, and tends to move in and out of the body more quickly, making repeated doses necessary in short periods to maintain pain relief.

Medication choice and dosing for PCA are extremely important and based on the individual. The patients must receive enough loading medication either through intermittent injection of doses via the PCA or through the IV so that the patient reaches a comfort level

Table 12.1 ■ *Medication Doses for Use in PCAs*

Medications	*Loading Dose*	*Bolus Dose*	*Lockout*
Morphine	2 mg	1–2 mg	6–10 min
Hydromorphone	0.5 mg	0.2–0.4 mg	6–10 min
Fentanyl	25 μg	10–20 mcg	5–10 min
Buprenorphine		0.03–0.1 mg	8–20 min
Methadone		0.5 mg	8–20 min
Meperidine: Not recommended for use			
Basal infusions not recommended for opioid-naïve patients.			

Sources: Grass, 2005; Hurley, Cohen, & Wu, 2010.

that can be maintained by bolus doses. Medications that can be used in PCA pumps include the following:

Morphine is considered the gold standard for IV PCA and equianalgesic conversions. Excreted by glucuronidation, it has a metabolite called morphine-6-glucuronide that is renally excreted, creating the potential for accumulation with delayed excretion. This increases the potential for increasing and delaying sedation in patients with renal impairment. Hydrophilic activity with maximum serum levels is reached within 6 minutes and a steady state is reached within 16 to 20 hours (Thomas & von Gunten, 2006).

Hydromorphone (Dilaudid) is considered 6 times more potent than morphine (Grass, 2005). It is metabolized in the liver and excreted as an inactive glucuronide metabolite, which is a benefit for patients with renal impairment. Small doses can provide a high level of pain relief, thus decreasing the potential for adverse effects, such as nausea or pruritis. The hydrophilic action is similar to morphine. Hydromorphone is more midrange than morphine and reaches peak effect in 30 minutes to 1 hour (Fine & Portenoy, 2007).

Fentanyl (Sublimaze) is considered 80–100 times more potent than morphine with single doses and, with repeated dosing, 33–40 times the potency of morphine (Grass, 2005). It is metabolized in the liver and is not renally excreted, making it a suitable medication for patients with renal failure. Its lipophilicity not only provides high bioavailability and can easily penetrate the blood-brain barrier but also has a rapid offset (Thomas & von Gunten, 2006). Peak effect is reached in less than 10 minutes (Fine & Portenoy, 2007).

Methadone (Dolophine) has lipophilic action with mu-receptor agonism coupled with *N*-methyl-d-aspartate (NMDA) receptor antagonist activity (Hurley, Cohen, & Wu, 2010). Prescribing should be reserved for pain specialists or those familiar with methadone prescribing and use should be confined to special patient populations, such as oncology patients. The half-life of methadone is 8 to 72 hours, with 1 to 15 days required to get to a steady state (Thomas & von Gunten, 2006). This time delay creates a significant potential for delayed respiratory depression (APS, 2008). Because of the extended half-life, it may be considered a good choice for highly opioid-tolerant oncology patients. Peak effect with methadone is variable but is generally considered to be within 1 to 2 hours (Fine & Portenoy, 2007). Extreme caution should be used in opioid-naïve patients. There is also a potential for cardiac arrhythmias with long-term use. Patients on high-dose medications will need an electrocardiogram (ECG) as a baseline at medication initiation and an ECG every 6 months to monitor for any Q-T interval changes (APS, 2008).

Buprenorphine (Buprenex) is a mixed agonist–antagonist activity mu-opioid receptor partial agonist coupled with kappa opioid receptor antagonist (Hurley, Cohen, & Wu, 2010). It is not considered a first-line option for pain relief, but it has been used successfully for gynecological surgeries. It may provoke an acute withdrawal syndrome when a pure opioid agonist has been used for pain control before the mixed agonist–antagonist. It also has a high potential for psychotomimetic side effects, such as hallucinations (Grass, 2005).

Ketamine is an NMDA-receptor antagonist that blocks activation of NMDA receptor sites that are activated with continued pain stimulus. Combined with opioids in PCA, low-dose ketamine has been shown to reduce opioid consumption (Subramaniam et al., 2004), but other studies have shown little to no effect on reducing pain, opioid consumption, or side effects (Hurley, Cohen, & Wu, 2010). Additionally, ketamine has a high profile for side effects, such as hallucinations, memory problems, abuse, and addiction (APS, 2008). Given the mixed results of the current studies, more research on ketamine use would need to have more consistently positive results to receive a positive clinical recommendation.

One medication that has fallen out of favor for use in general pain management as well as PCAs is meperidine (Demerol). For many years, meperidine was a mainstay for pain relief in postoperative patients. Now, pain management societies have moved the medication from a first-line pain medication to a second-line option and discourage its use altogether. Meperidine has the potential for seizures associated with a toxic metabolite called normeperidine that can accumulate in the central nervous system (CNS) fluid. For these reasons, it is not recommended for use with patients who have a renal impairment or CNS disease. It should not be for long-term use and if used at all, the cumulative daily dose should be no higher than 600 mg/day, and it should be used for the shortest time possible. The best choice is to avoid use of this medication and select one of the other medications, such as morphine or hydromorphone, for PCA use.

The Joint Commission recommends that all hospitals have standard or preprinted orders that can be used by any practitioners licensed to prescribe opioids. Listed on the order set should be the drug, concentration, loading dose, bolus or demand dose, PCA lockout, and 1- or 4-hour totals. The Joint Commission also recommends the use of standardized concentrations so that fewer medication errors are made when unusual or nonstandard concentrations are ordered. Included on the order set should be a monitoring protocol for frequency of vital signs, oxygen saturation, and respiratory status. Some order sets include an order for naloxone (Narcan), an opioid reversal agent that is used to reverse oversedation in patients. An additional section listing treatments for adverse effects such as nausea/vomiting, pruritis, and urinary retention should be included.

Setting up a PCA requires a knowledge of the patient's opioid use prior to the surgery, any prior difficulties with particular opioids, and a knowledge of what medications are commonly used for PCA. The use of a basal rate on PCA, where medication that is continuously delivered is not recommended for opioid-naïve patients (Acute Pain Management Scientific Evidence, 2005; APS, 2008; Grass, 2005; Hurley, Cohen, & Wu, 2010; Institute for Safe Medication Practice [ISMP], 2009). It has been found to have little additive effect for pain relief, but it is considered to be a high-risk factor for increasing sedation (APS, 2008; ISMP, 2009). The use of basal infusions on PCA is more appropriate; in fact, it is a necessity when highly opioid-tolerant patients are not taking oral medications and need to have their usual daily oral medication dose changed to PCA delivery postoperatively.

To order a PCA for a patient, first select the opioid with a standard concentration, select the doses and lockout, and add any additional orders for antiemetics, laxative doses, and so forth. For example, a PCA prescription might read the following:

Drug—Morphine 1 mg/ml
Mode—PCA only—no basal rate selected
Loading dose: 2 mg
Dose: 1 mg
Lockout 6 min
1 hour total: 10 mg
Clinician bolus: 2 mg every 4 hours as needed for increased pain or activity; no more than four doses in a 24-hour period
Monitoring parameters, respiratory rate, oxygenation, vital signs, and so forth
Laxatives, antiemetics

An example of a standardized order sheet is provided in Figure 12.1.

Other important elements of PCA ordering to consider are the following:

- The loading doses for morphine should be patient dependent and range between 2 and 4 mg (Grass, 2005). An equianalgesic conversion can be used to order loading doses with other medications (e.g., hydromorphone [0.4 to 0.8 mg]).
- The 1- or 4-hour total is controversial at this time. There are differing opinions as to the necessity of the parameter or whether a 1- or 4-hour total is more effective. The advantage to using a 1-hour total, which should equal the total number of doses available to the patient in the hour, is that you can quickly determine if there is a need for adjusting PCA doses. By waiting 4 hours, the patients may be underdosed or overdosed for a longer period.

Patient Controlled Analgesia (PCA)
PHYSICIAN'S ORDERS

ALLERGIES ➤ ☐ NKDA ☐ Other ____________

I HEREBY AUTHORIZE THE PHARMACY TO DISPENSE A GENERIC EQUIVALENT UNLESS THE PARTICULAR DRUG IS CIRCLED.

PATIENT PLATE

Physicians: Please draw a line through any orders not desired.

Patient Controlled Analgesia (PCA) Standard Physician Orders

Discontinue all opioids or sedatives unless ordered for use WITH PCA by MD writing PCA orders.

☐ IV Fluid ____________ (solution) at ________ ml/hr.

☐ Analgesic: ☐ Morphine 1 mg/ml ☐ Dilaudid 1 mg/ml ☐ Fentanyl 12.5 **micrograms**/ml.

☐ Method of administration:
☐ IV PCA only ☐ IV CONTINUOUS only ☐ IV PCA and CONTINUOUS

☐ Medication to be administered via PCA pump: (indicate **milligrams** or **micrograms**)
LOADING DOSE (optional): __________ ☐ **mg** ☐ **micrograms** (by pump)
(Suggested adult morphine 2 mg, Dilaudid 0.5 mg., Fentanyl 25 **micrograms**)

CONTINUOUS INFUSION (optional): __________ ☐ **mg** or ☐ **micrograms** per hour
(suggested adult Morphine 1 mg/h., Dilaudid 0.2 mg/h., Fentanyl 12.5 **micrograms**/h)
*Caution for elderly > 65 y of age, or opioid naïve patients

ON DEMAND DOSE (PCA dose): __________ ☐ **mg** or ☐ **micrograms**
(suggested starting adult dose Morphine 1 mg., Dilaudid 0.2 mg., Fentanyl 12.5 **micrograms**)

LOCKOUT INTERVAL: __________ minutes (suggested 6 or 8 minutes)

1 HOUR LIMIT (Maximum amount of drug in **1** hour. Should equal total amount of hourly doses.)
__________ ☐ **mg** or ☐ **micrograms**
(suggested adult Morphine 10 mg., Dilaudid 3 mg., Fentanyl 200 **micrograms**)

☐ **Clinician bolus:** For increased pain or pain related to increased activity, nurse may bolus patient with selected medication above ____ ☐ **mg** or ☐ **micrograms** every ______ hours. No more than 4 doses in a 24 hour period.

☐ In case of IV failure and inability to restart IV give ____________ ☐ SQ ☐ IM ☐ PO every ______ hour prn and call physician.

☐ Assessment: Documented on the Pain Documentation Sheet.
***Vital signs, O2 saturation and sedation level** every 15 minutes x 4 at start and then every ____ hrs and each time analgesic dose is increased.
*For **respirations** less than 8 per minute, stop PCA pump.
- Narcan Administration:
  1. Dilute one amp of Narcan (0.4 mg.) in 10 ml of normal saline.
  2. Once Narcan is diluted as above:
     For **unarousable** patients give 2.5 ml (0.1mg.) slow IV push. If no response in 90 seconds repeat dose.
     For **apneic patients or resp. rate < 4 per minute** give 5 ml (0.2 mg.) of diluted Narcan solution slow IV push. If no response after 90 seconds repeat dose. Continue to repeat dose until resp. rate > 14 or O2 saturation 94% or greater.

*Get **STAT ABGs** oxygen saturation and apply O2 at 2 liters nasal cannula for saturation less than 94%.
*Notify Pain Specialist for all occurrences of sedation requiring Narcan administration - send computer consult.

☐ Antiemetic: ______ ____ mg ☐ IV ☐ IM ☐ PO ☐ Rectal every ____ hrs prn nausea/vomiting

☐ Laxative: __________ ____ (dose) every ______ hr ☐ PO ☐ Rectal PRN constipation.

SIGNATURE TITLE DATE TIME PRINTED | SIGNATURE TITLE DATE TIME PRINTED

PATIENT SAFETY ALERT

USE	Do not use
DAILY	QD
EVERY OTHER DAY	QOD
UNITS	U
0.5 MG.	Lack of leading zero (e.g. .5 mg)
10 MG.	Trailing zero (e.g. 10.0 mg)
MORPHINE SULFATE	MS or MSO4
MAGNESIUM SULFATE	MgSO4
MICRO-GRAM OR MCG.	µg or µ for microgram
INTER-NATIONAL UNITS	IU
LEFT EAR; RIGHT EAR; BOTH EARS	A.S.; A.D.; A.U.
LEFT EYE; RIGHT EYE; BOTH EYES;	O.S.; O.D.; O.U.

Figure 12.1 ■ PCA order set exemplar. *Source:* Courtesy of Suburban Hospital–Johns Hopkins Medicine, Bethesda, MD.

- Using clinician or supplemental boluses allows the nurse to give an extra dose of medication when the patient needs it. For example, if a patient falls asleep and does not push the button and wakes in pain, the nurse can administer the extra dose after assessing that the patient is stable enough to tolerate the additional medication. These doses are also helpful for providing the patients with additional medication for activity such as physical therapy or walking around the unit.

Monitoring parameters helps to ensure that the patient is being carefully watched while using PCA. If supplemental oxygen is being used, electronic monitoring with pulse oximetry may be skewed with blood oxygen levels in the 70s, although oximetry readings may be much higher (Vila, 2005). Having the nurse assess the patient regularly every 2 to 4 hours can provide a trained eye on the patient's real status.

Additionally, capnography has been found to provide a more accurate reading on blood oxygen levels in postoperative patients and is being used more frequently in the postoperative setting to detect increasing CO_2 levels that could lead to oversedation. Some PCA pumps have an in-line capnography system that can monitor CO_2 levels while the PCA is being used.

Monitoring Patient-Controlled Analgesia and Treating Adverse Effects With Patient-Controlled Analgesia

Sedation/Oversedation

Respiratory depression, sedation, and oversedation can occur with any patient. Although these events are thought to occur frequently, the actual level of occurrence is thought to be less than 5% (Hurley, Cohen, & Wu, 2010), from 0.19% to 5.2% (Hagle, Lehr, Brubakken, & Shippee, 2004), or 0.25% (Grass, 2005). Compared with the incidence of respiratory depression of 0.9% for IM injections, the PCA compares favorably (Grass, 2005). Monitoring parameters are set by order on the PCA form. Using a simple numeric sedation scale, the Ramsay on general nursing units or the Richmond Agitation Sedation

Scale (RASS) in critical settings, may find early stages of sedation and avoid progression to oversedation. Conditions that contribute to respiratory depression with PCA use include concomitant administration of other sedating agents, such as sleeping medications, the use of a basal rate, advanced age, and pulmonary conditions, such as sleep apnea (Hurley, Cohen, & Wu, 2010). Additionally, Hagle et al. (2004) report that risk factors for sedation with PCA include being over the age of 70 years; basal infusion with IV PCA; renal, hepatic, pulmonary, or cardiac impairment; sleep apnea; concurrent CNS depressants; obesity; upper abdominal or thoracic surgery; and an IV PCA bolus dose greater than 1 mg.

If the patient becomes oversedated, the use of naloxone (Narcan) is recommended to reverse the effects of the opioid and restore normal respiratory status. If Narcan is administered, an alternate form of pain management will be needed in the immediate postadministration period. For patients with sleep apnea, the American Society of Anesthesiologists (ASA) and The Joint Commission recommend more aggressive monitoring when opioids are used in the postoperative setting.

Postoperative Nausea and Vomiting

All opioid medications have the potential to create nausea and vomiting. A consensus guideline by the ASA (2004) indicates that some patients have higher risk factors for postoperative nausea and vomiting (PONV), including female sex, history of motion sickness or PONV, nonsmoker, and use of postoperative opioids. The use of antiemetics, such as ondansetron, is needed for these patients to control PONV. For many patients, the use of antiemetics starts in the operating room in an effort to control PONV.

Constipation

As with PONV, constipation is a natural outcome of regular opioid use. For all patients using opioids for postoperative pain control, laxatives and stool softeners are recommended to maintain adequate bowel function. Constipation is the only adverse effect for which patients cannot become tolerant. The use of stool softeners, such as docusate (Colace), and laxatives, such as senna (Senokot), polyethylene glycol 3350 (MiraLAX), or Milk of Magnesia, can restore normal bowel function despite opioid use.

Pruritis

All opioids can cause pruritis, and some patients are more prone to pruritis with opioids. The occurrence of pruritis does not mean that the patient has an allergy to the medications. The generalized itching felt by a patient with opioid use is thought to be the result of histamine release or another unknown physiologic mechanism. It follows, therefore, that the use of an antihistamine such as diphenhydramine (Benadryl) is recommended. Unfortunately, if diphenhydramine is used, it can add to the cumulative sedation potential for the patients and lower doses are considered appropriate, especially if it is used for the elderly. One medication used to reduce pruritis is nalbuphine (Nubain) at a dose one fourth to one half of the standard dose, 2.5 to 5 mg IV, but the health care provider should be aware that this is an off-label medication use.

Delirium and Confusion

For older patients taken out of familiar surroundings and receiving medications for pain and surgery, confusion and delirium can occur. Some practitioners confuse the demented patient's progressive decline in cognitive function with delirium, a sudden onset of an acute confusional state. Although most often considered a condition that affects the older patient, delirium can happen to any patient who receives opioids or surgical medications, or who undergoes a form of sedation. The incidence of delirium in the general hospital population is felt to range from 10% to 60% of all patients (Vaurio, Sande, Wang, Mullen, & Leung, 2006). Patients who are taking oral pain medications have less delirium, whereas those patients who are older and those who receive IV pain medications have a higher rate of delirium (Vaurio et al., 2006). It is also important to note that unrelieved pain can contribute to delirium. If a patient on PCA becomes confused, changing medication to the oral route may help, but adding other nonopioid interventions, such as NSAIDs, blocks, and neural blockade, may be helpful while eliminating other contributing medications, such as benzodiazepines and other medications with CNS effects.

Recommendations for Safe Patient-Controlled Analgesia Use

The Joint Commission and the ISMP have tracked PCA use for many years. They have found that there are significant safety issues with PCA and have issued some recommendations to make the practice safer for all prescribers and patients.

One of the issues that have emerged from safety monitoring systems includes cases of overdose and death with PCA, with the PCA found to play a role in each case (ISMP, 2003; The Joint Commission, 2005). Current estimates of risk with PCA indicate that death from user programming errors was 1 in 33,000 to 1 in 338,800, resulting in an estimated 65 to 667 deaths in the history of use of the device (Vicente, Kada-Bekhaled, Hillel, Cassano, & Orser, 2003). Other concerns are linked to operator error and misprogramming. In one quality improvement study, 71% of the errors found were related to misprogramming causing either overmedication or undermedication, 15% were related to human factors resulting in the administration of the wrong medication, and 9% were related to equipment problems (Weir, 2005).

Breaking down the programming errors, the most common errors were found to include the following:

- Confusion over milliliter and milligram
- Confusing the PCA bolus dose with the basal dose
- Entering the loading dose instead of the bolus dose
- Wrong lockout setting selected
- Wrong medication concentration selected (ISMP, 2003)

Because of the errors that were found in the monitoring systems, The Joint Commission and ISMP have made recommendations about PCA that can help to ensure the safest possible PCA practice. The current recommendations include two independent nurse checks of medication, concentration, and dose settings; clear identification of the IV line where the PCA is infusing; use of prefilled syringes or bags; and use of standardized order sets.

The Joint Commission has also addressed some pertinent practice issues and has made recommendations for practice in these areas.

Proper Patient Selection

Each organization using PCA for analgesia should have a group of patients who are good candidates for PCA and a group of patients who are not good candidates for PCA use. Choosing the correct patient type and limiting PCA use to those patients who are good candidates can ensure that PCA is properly used. PCA is a fairly simple concept to understand, and children as young as 5 years of age have demonstrated that they can safely activate a PCA pump. The Joint Commission and ISMP have listed several patient groups that they feel are not good candidates for PCA use, including infants and young children; confused older adults; patients who are obese or have sleep apnea or asthma; and patients taking other medications with sedating effects, such as muscle relaxants, antiemetics, and sleeping medications (Cohen & Smetzer, 2005).

Patient-Controlled Analgesia by Proxy

The term PCA by proxy is usually defined as the activation of the PCA pump by someone other than the patient, usually a friend or family member who perceives the patient to be in pain but unable to activate the pump independently. Most hospitals have a policy that prevents anyone but the patient from activating the PCA. This prohibition includes nurses or other staff members. Once the patient is removed from the PCA process, the potential for potentially fatal oversedation is very real. Of the 460 PCA errors reported to the PCA errors database of the United States Pharmacopeia, 12 were related to PCA by proxy with 1 fatal event. In some pediatric settings, hospitals have a set of rules and regulations that allow family members to activate the button for a child but the guidelines provided must be strictly observed to maintain patient safety.

Patient-Controlled Analgesia Pump Safety

Because the PCA pump is an integral piece of the PCA process, safe pump design can help to minimize the occurrence of adverse events, medication errors, and misprogramming. PCA pump buttons should not resemble call lights so that the patient can determine which button brings the nurse and which one delivers pain medication. Intuitive programming features can make it easier for nurses to enter prescriptions and to monitor medication usage. Free flow protection should be a part of every pump that is designed for use as a PCA.

Human Errors

Human errors are always possible when interacting with machines, but designing pumps that are simple and easy to use while protecting the patient can help to decrease error. Nurses are also responsible for learning to correctly enter PCA orders and maintaining competency in PCA practice. Using root cause analysis after PCA-related incidents can help pinpoint areas in the PCA process that need correction so that future errors can be avoided.

Patients Needing Special Consideration With Patient-Controlled Analgesia Use

Although The Joint Commission has set recommendations for patient selection with PCA use, there are other patient populations that require special consideration. Cognitively intact older patients, patients with a history of substance abuse, and patients who use opioids for relief of chronic pain require special consideration when PCA is being considered as a means of pain control. Other factors, such as weight, play no role in PCA dosing, although men have been found to require more morphine than women (Burns et al., 1989).

Older Patients

Patients who are older than 65 years require special considerations when PCA is being used for pain management. Despite the older age, they can be excellent candidates for PCA use, especially during large orthopedic procedures, such as total joint replacements. Most of these patients are opioid naïve and have some level of organ dysfunction related to age. For these patients, opioids can be prescribed, but the doses should be reduced by 25% to 50% and monitoring should be more frequent. In a study comparing morphine consumption in younger versus older patients, for patients 20 to 30 years of age, morphine consumption was 75 mg, whereas for those patients 60 to 70 years of age, the morphine consumption was 30 mg (Macintyre & Jarvis, 1996). Older age seems to be an indicator that less pain medication may be needed to control pain.

Patients With Chronic Pain

Patients who have chronic pain or who are taking regular opioids for pain relief are another difficult-to-treat patient group. These patients have increased pain-processing pathophysiology that may make their pain more intense, may increase sensitivity to pain, and may reduce effectiveness of opioids. For these patients, they will require their normal daily doses of opioids to be restarted as soon as possible and continued through their hospitalization. They will also need additional medication for the new acute pain above and beyond their usual daily opioid requirements. If the usual oral medications cannot be restarted in a timely fashion, the conversion to IV or PCA will need to be made, but the efficacy of these doses may also be reduced. For these patients, a continuous infusion using an equianalgesic conversion and allowing for the PCA demand dose medication will have to be performed. Many pharmacists are skilled at these conversions and are willing to help the prescriber with conversion doses.

Patients With a Substance Abuse History

For patients with a history of substance abuse or active drug use, treating pain either from acute injury or surgery is a challenge. Because there is no equianalgesic conversion or quality control for street drugs, a best guess estimate will be needed and a full history of how much drug is being used daily is essential. Actively addicted patients will need a continuous infusion with generous bolus doses to account for any underdosing.

Patients with a history of substance abuse are those who have used drugs in the past; however, although they are not using them now, they still have pathophysiologic changes that make treating the pain more difficult. They also have an increased sensitivity to pain stimulus and a decreased efficacy of opioid medications. For these patients, a continuous rate may be needed, and the doses will need to be higher than the surgery or acute pain might indicate. Although these patients are highly opioid tolerant, it is still possible to have them become oversedated if the doses are large enough, so it is important to maintain the frequent monitoring parameters.

For all of these patients, PCA is a good option, although there are adjustments that will need to be made. It is important to set up reasonable expectations about medication use and pain relief. Postoperative patients cannot expect to be pain free, and although some patients have chronic pain, the focus in the postoperative setting is on surgical pain. Adequate postoperative pain management should facilitate activity, restore functional status, and provide for a timely discharge.

Clinical Pearl

To use the 0 to 10 NPS for difficult-to-treat patients, ask the patient with chronic pain what his or her average daily pain score is and set a realistic pain goal of 2 or 3 points lower for the new acute pain. For older patients, set an achievable pain goal and ask the patient what pain rating would be reasonable to participate in activity and physical therapy. For addicted patients or patients with a history of substance abuse, set parameters around medication use and set a reasonable goal for pain relief. Explain that no pain or 0/10 pain is not reasonable for the type of surgery/injury the patient has sustained. Also indicate that purposeful sedation is not the goal of PCA therapy, but rather it is the pain relief that is the focus and goal.

Case Study

Jane Jones is a 45-year-old patient who has just had a total abdominal hysterectomy. She is using a Dilaudid PCA set at 0.2 mg, 10 min/1.2 mg, 1 hour total for postoperative pain relief. She is still NPO and is only allowed ice chips. In her preoperative history, she reports having diabetes, painful diabetic neuropathy, and a history of migraine headaches. She reports taking Oxycontin, 20 mg every 12 hours, Vicodin, two tablets every 6 hours as needed for breakthrough pain, a medication for migraines when needed, and a naturopathic pain medication. She states she has been taking her Vicodin regularly for her abdominal and back pain prior to her surgery.

Postoperatively, Jane complains of unrelieved pain and stops using her PCA pump. When asked why she has stopped pushing the button, she replies that when she does use the PCA, it does nothing for her pain. She refuses to ambulate and complains of postoperative nausea. How can we improve Jane's pain management?

Questions to Consider

1. What would be the first option for improving Jane's pain management: changing medications, changing doses, or changing lockout?
2. Should Jane have her oral medications restarted? If not, is the equianalgesic conversion of her current PCA settings enough to control her new pain and chronic underlying pain conditions?
3. Should we consider additional pain medications under interventional option?
4. Is Jane at risk for delirium, constipation, or other side effects of opioid use? If so, what types of options can be used to resolve the effects?
5. Does Jane fall into any of the high-risk categories that The Joint Commission has identified for PCA use? Should we ask her about her preoperative pain levels?

REFERENCES

Acute Pain Management: SE Working Group of the Australian and New Zealand College of Anaesthetists and Faculty of Pain Medicine. (2005). *Acute pain management: Scientific evidence* (2nd ed.). Melbourne, Australia: Authors.

American Pain Society. (2008). *Principles of analgesic use in the treatment of acute pain and cancer pain* (6th ed.). Glenview, IL: Author.

American Society of Anesthesiologists. (2004). *Practice guidelines for acute pain management in the perioperative setting*. Park Ridge, IL: Author.

Burns, J. W., Hodsman, N. B. A., McLintock, T. T. C., Gillies, G. W. A., Kenny, G. N. C., & McArdle, C. S. (1989). The influence of patient characteristics on the requirements for postoperative analgesia. *Anaesthesia*, *44*(1), 2–6.

Cohen, M. R., & Smetzer, J. (2005). Patient-controlled analgesia safety issues. *Journal of Pain and Palliative Care Pharmacotherapy, 19*(1), 45–50.

D'Arcy, Y. (2007). Manage pain across the perioperative spectrum. *OR Nurse, 1*(3), 38–42.

D'Arcy, Y. (2008a). First strike: Does preemptive analgesia work? *Nursing, 38*(4), 52–55.

D'Arcy, Y. (2008b). Keep your patient safe during PCA. *Nursing, 38*(1), 50–55.

Fine, P., & Portenoy, R. (2007). *A clinical guide to opioid analgesia.* New York, NY: Vendome Group LLC.

Gan, T. J., Meyer, T., Apfel, C. C., Chung, F., Davis, P. J., Eubanks, S., Kovac, A., & Watcha, M. (2003). Department of Anesthesiology, Duke University Medical Center. Consensus guidelines for managing postoperative nausea and vomiting. *Anesthesia and Analgesia, 97,* 62–71.

Grass, J. A. (2005). Patient-controlled analgesia. *Anesthesia and Analgesia, 101,* S44–S61.

Hagle, M., Lehr, V. T., Brubakken, K., & Shippee, A. (2004). Respiratory depression in adult patients with intravenous patient-controlled analgesia. *Orthopaedic Nursing, 23*(1), 18–27.

Hudcova, J., McNicol, E. D., Quah, C. S., Lau, J., & Carr, D. B. (2006). Patient-controlled opioid analgesia versus conventional opioid analgesia for postoperative pain. *Cochrane Database of Systematic Reviews* (4), CD003348.

Hurley, R. W., Cohen, S. P., & Wu, C. L. (2010). Acute pain in adults. In S. Fishman, J. Ballantyne, & J. Rathmell (Eds.), *Bonica's management of pain* (4th ed., pp. 699–706). Philadelphia, PA: Wolters Kluwer Health/Lippincott Williams & Wilkins.

Institute for Safe Medication Practices. (2003). *Patient-controlled analgesia: Making it safer for patients.* Retrieved from www.ismp.org/profdevelopment/PCA Monograph.pdf

Institute for Safe Medication Practices Medication Safety Alert. (2009). Beware of basal opioid infusions with PCA therapy. *Nurse Advis-ERR, 7*(10). Retrieved from http://www.ismp.org/Newsletters/nursing/issues

The Joint Commission. (2004). Patient-controlled analgesia by proxy. *Sentinel Events Alert, 33.*

The Joint Commission. (2005). Focus on five: Preventing patient-controlled analgesia overdose. *Joint Commission Perspective on Patient Safety, 5*(10), 11–11(1).

Macintyre, P. E., & Jarvis, D. A. (1996). Age is the best predictor of post-operative morphine requirements. *Pain, 64*(2), 357–364.

Subramaniam, K., Subramaniam, B., & Steinbrook, R. A. (2004). Ketamine as adjuvant analgesic to opioids: A quantitative and qualitative systematic review. *Anesthesia & Analgesia, 99*(2), 482–495.

Thomas, J., & von Gunten, C. (2006). Pharmacologic therapies for pain. In J. Von Roenn, J. Paice, M. E. Preodor, & M. Lange (Eds.), *Current diagnosis & treatment of pain* (pp. 21–37). New York: McGraw-Hill.

Vaurio, L. E., Sande, L. P., Wang, Y., Mullen, E. A., & Leung, J. M. (2006). Postoperative delirium: The importance of pain and pain management. *Anesthesia and Analgesia*, *102*(4), 1267–1273.

Vicente, K. J., Kada-Bekhaled, K., Hillel, G., Cassano, A., & Orser, B. A. (2003). Programming errors contribute to death from patient-controlled analgesia: Case report and estimate of probability. *Canadian Journal of Anaesthesia*, *50*, 328–332.

Vila, H., Jr., Smith, R. A., Augustyniak, M. J., Nagi, P. A., Soto, R. G., Ross, T. W., . . . Miguel, R. V. (2005). The efficacy and safety of pain management before and after implementation of hospital-wide pain management standards: Is patient safety compromised by treatment based solely on numerical pain ratings? *Anesthesia & Analgesia*, *101*(2), 474–480.

Weir, V. L. (2005). Best practice protocols: Preventing adverse drug events. *Nursing Management*, *36*(9), 24–30.

13

Epidural Analgesia

EPIDURAL BASICS

Epidural pain management can provide the largest amount of pain relief with the least amount of medication. This is because equianalgesically, the doses of opioids delivered to the epidural and intrathecal spaces are several times more potent than the same medications given intravenously. Adding a local anesthetic, such as bupivacaine or ropivacaine, to the epidural solution creates a synergistic effect that enhances the overall analgesic effect of the epidural.

In most cases, the epidural analgesia is administered perioperatively and either used during surgery as an alternate to general anesthesia or used not only during surgery but also as postoperative analgesia. The opioid medications used for epidural pain management bind to opioid receptors in the dorsal horn of the spinal cord and can produce effective analgesia at greatly reduced doses. The addition of local anesthetic allows the nerve roots closest to the placement site to be bathed in the epidural solution, causing localized pain relief. In most cases, epidurals used for postoperative pain relief have solutions that contain both low-dose opioids and local anesthetic.

Some patients are resistant to epidural catheters, fearing that they will have a needle in their back during the time of the infusion. Patients should be reassured that the needle is only used for placing the catheter, and the tubing that remains is very small and soft.

Patients who are good candidates for epidural analgesia are patients with major surgeries that include:

- Thoracotomy
- Large abdominal surgeries
- Aortic aneurysm repair
- Orthopedic surgery (e.g., total joint replacements)
- Labor and delivery (e.g., used for delivery)
- Surgery for multiple rib fractures or flail chest (e.g., Level 1; Evidence from Guidelines for Blunt Force Trauma, 2004)

To place an epidural catheter, the patient is placed into a sitting position or side lying position with the back flexed in an outward curve. The anesthesiologist or certified nurse anesthetist inserts a beveled hollow needle through the skin of the back into the epidural space, which is really a potential space between the ligament flavum and the dura mater. Once the fluid enters the epidural space, it expands, much like blowing air into a flat paper bag. Once the needle is placed at the correct dermatome, the epidural catheter is threaded through the needle and placement is confirmed by a technique called *loss of resistance*. This means that there is a decreased resistance to preservative-free sterile saline being pushed through the catheter once it reaches the open area of the epidural space (see Figure 13.1). For epidural placement, the needle itself does not extend into the cerebrospinal fluid (CSF) or the spinal cord.

Once the anesthesiologist or certified nurse anesthetist feels a loss of resistance, he or she is fairly certain that the epidural space has been entered. After the catheter is determined to be placed properly, the practitioner can then bolus the catheter to determine the effect. The epidural space contains various structures that include spinal nerve roots, fat, areolar tissue, lymph tissue, and blood vessels, including a rich venous plexus (Rockford & DeRuyter, 2009). Because the analgesic effect is so localized, the catheter is placed at the level of the expected surgical incision, with catheter placement being done commonly in the thoracic and lumbar spinal levels. The medication "spread" is determined by the site of injection. Spread is defined as the spread of the medication, either rostral

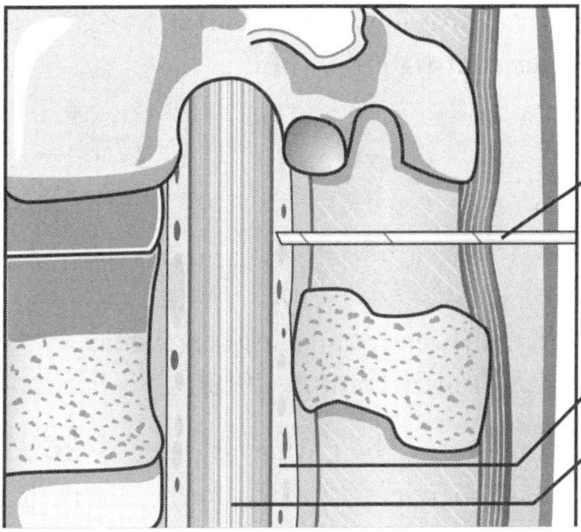

Figure 13.1 ■ The epidural space

(upward) or caudal (downward) from the expected dermatomal level. Additional factors that may influence the spread of the medication are the patient's age and volume of drug being infused (Rockford & DeRuyter, 2009).

It is important to note that once the epidural catheter reaches the epidural space, it can migrate in a rostral or caudal direction. This migration can affect the way the patient feels analgesic effect. In some cases, the epidural catheter provides analgesia to a nonoperative lower extremity when the intent is to provide analgesia to the operative extremity. This effect is caused by the curling of the catheter in the epidural space, leading to a reduced effect in the desired location.

Spinal or Intrathecal Differences

The term *spinal* can be used for either epidural or intrathecal analgesia, but it is more precise to use the terms epidural and intrathecal, although the term spinal is closely associated with intrathecal placement. For some patients, a single dose of preservative-free morphine is used as an adjunct for postoperative analgesia. These doses are commonly referred to as *single shots*. They are given one time only, and an extended-release morphine, such as Astramorph, Duramorph, or DepoDur, is used to extend the action of the medication for 24 hours. Because morphine is a hydrophilic medication, it can spread throughout the CSF and extend the action of the medication. A single-shot Duramorph injection is done using 0.1 to 0.3 mg, with the dose being dependent on the patient's history and prior opioid use (American Pain Society [APS], 2008).

When an intrathecal catheter is placed for continuous infusion, the catheter extends directly into the intrathecal space (see Figure 13.2) and the medications flow into the CSF fluid. Either opioids or local anesthetics can be used intrathecally, but continuous

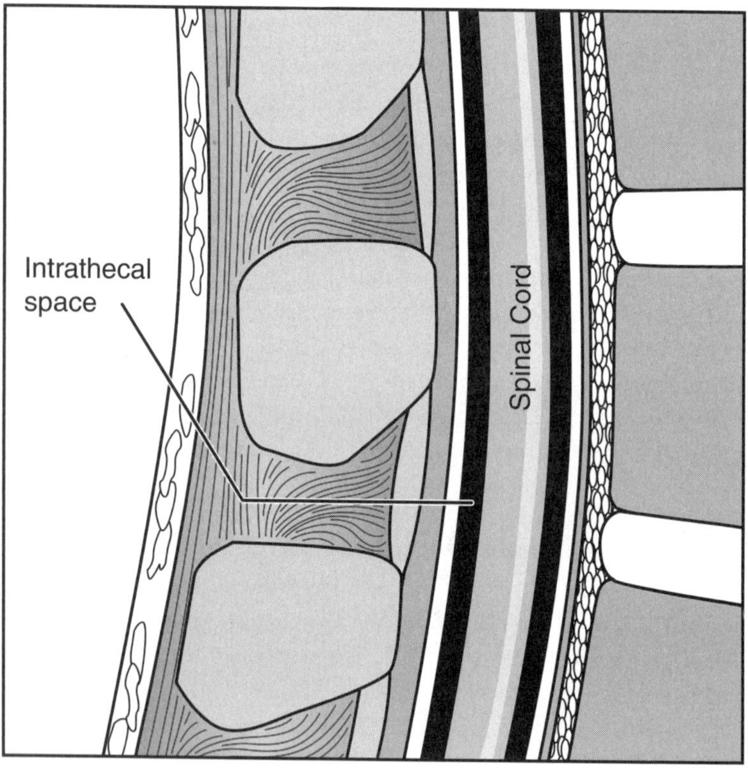

Figure 13.2 ■ The intrathecal space

infusion of local anesthetics are associated in some cases with the development of cauda equina syndrome (Acute Pain: Scientific Evidence, 2005). A combined spinal (intrathecal)-epidural technique can provide a faster onset of analgesia and increased maternal satisfaction with pain relief during labor (Hughes, Simmons, & Brown, 2003).

Because medications that are inserted into the epidural space need to cross the dura, the onset of action with epidural analgesia is slower when compared with intrathecal administration. Because medications infused into the intrathecal space spread through the CSF, a hydrophilic medication, such as a morphine, is more useful. Uptake can take place locally at the site of the insertion through spinal blood vessels, fatty tissue, and CSF, and doses lower than those used epidurally may produce effective analgesia.

Epidural Medications

All medications used for epidural analgesia should be preservative free because many preservatives, such as alcohol-based preparations, can damage neural tissue. The opioid medications used for epidural analgesia are basically the same as those used with patient-controlled analgesia (PCA), but there are also different local anesthetic agents that are used in combined solutions. When epidural medications are compared with intrathecal medication administration, the epidural route has fewer side effects and a lessened potential for respiratory depression (Rockford & DeRuyter, 2009).

Opioids

Morphine, hydromorphone (Dilaudid), and fentanyl (Sublimaze) are the three most common medications used for epidural analgesia (Table 13.1). The two drugs recommended for use in epidurals are morphine and fentanyl, with hydromophone having less evidence for use (American Society of Anesthesiologists [ASA] Task Force on Acute Pain Management, 2004). The choice of which medication to use for infusion is provider dependent and patient specific. If the

Table 13.1 ■ *Medications Used for Epidural Infusions*

Medication	*Loading Dose*	*Continuous Infusion*	*Bolus Dose (PCEA)*	*Lockout*	*Onset*	*Duration of Single Dose*
Morphine	1–6 mg (age dependent)	0.1–1.0 mg/hr	50–200 mcg[a]	30–45 min	30 min	6–24 hours
Fentanyl	50–100 mcg	50–100 mcg/hr	15–20 mcg	10 min	5 min	4–8 hours
Hydromorphone	0.4–1.0 mg	30–120 mcg/hr	20–40 mcg	15 min	5–8 min	4–6 hours
Clonidine[b]	NA	0.30	NA	NA	NA	NA
Local Anesthetic						
Bupivacaine 0.1%		3–10 ml/hr				
Ropivacaine 0.2%		3–10 ml/hr				

[a]NR, not recommended due to delay of action.
[b]Clonidine used as an adjuvant.
Source: APS, 2008; Rockford & DeRuyter, 2009.

patient has allergies to morphine, another medication is selected and adequate pain relief is the measure of effectiveness.

When comparing the use of morphine versus fentanyl, the pharmacokinetics show a differentiation of action. Morphine is a hydrophilic medication. When morphine is used in epidural solutions, there is a rapid rise in morphine serum concentration, and the action is similar to intravenous (IV) PCA (Rockford & DeRuyter, 2009). Conversely, when fentanyl, a lipophilic medication, is used in epidural solutions, the serum concentration of the medication rises more slowly because of medication uptake by epidural fat and other epidural tissues. To approximate the action of IV medication administration, it takes about 25 hours for the lipid uptake of fentanyl to allow the drug to freely enter the circulatory system (Rockford & DeRuyter, 2009). Morphine has a naturally occurring, longer action, whereas fentanyl has a shorter period of activity, making it more suitable for use as epidural PCA called patient-controlled epidural analgesia (PCEA) (APS, 2008). Hydromorphone is a midrange medication whose action falls somewhere between morphine and fentanyl.

Clinical Pearl

To compare equivalent doses of morphine, consider that morphine 30 mg orally is equivalent to 10 mg IV, 1 mg epidural, and 100 mcg intrathecal (APS, 2008).

Local Anesthetics

The two most commonly used local anesthetics (LA) for epidurals are preservative-free bupivacaine and ropivacaine. These medications are used because of all possible local anesthetics, they have the longest action, which makes them more suitable for continuous infusion. When used in an epidural solution, the role of the LA is to bathe the nerve roots, dorsal root ganglia, spinal nerves in the paravertebral space, and nerve rootlets, thus creating paresthesia and analgesia. Combining an LA with an opioid produces a synergistic effect and superior pain relief (Acute Pain: Scientific Evidence, 2005;

APS, 2008; Hurley, Cohen, & Wu, 2010). Ropivacaine is thought to have a lessened effect on muscles and is commonly used in epidurals for patients who will be actively engaged in physical therapy or early ambulation postoperatively, such as patients undergoing total joint replacement.

Additional Medications

Clonidine (Catapres-TTS) is an alpha-2 agonist used to treat pain. For neuropathic pain, a continuous infusion of clonidine at 30 mcg/h demonstrated positive effects (Eisenach, DuPen, Dubois, Miguel, & Allin, 1995). Other studies demonstrate an analgesic effect when clonidine is used alone and a synergistic effect to prolong epidural blockade (Forster & Rosenberg, 2004). Side effects of clonidine include hypotension, sedation, and bradycardia (Hurley et al, 2010). To stop a clonidine infusion, careful downward titration over several days is recommended to avoid rebound hypertension (Rockford & DeRuyter, 2009).

Monitoring Patients on Epidural Analgesia

Careful and consistent monitoring of patients with epidural analgesia is needed not only to ensure adequate analgesic but also to ensure the safety of patients using this method for postoperative pain relief. Vital signs, respiratory rates, and pain assessments will need to be done very frequently in the postoperative recovery unit and then hourly for the first few hours. Assessments can move to 2 hours after the initial postoperative period and then as the patient stabilizes.

Indicators that should be monitored include the following:

Site Care—Inspect the site for swelling, drainage, infiltration, and any signs of redness. The dressing over the epidural site should remain dry and intact. Tubing connections should be secured and remain tight (ASPMN, 2009).

Pain Relief—The patient's level of analgesia should be assessed regularly and dose adjustment made as needed with the order of the anesthesiologist. Patients may need bolus doses after physical activity or dose increase may be needed as postoperative medications wear off.

Other elements that should be assessed regularly include the following:

Respiratory Depression—Reduce or stop the opioid infusion. For significant sedation and decreased respiratory rate less than 8 or 10 breaths per minute, naloxone (Narcan) administration may be needed, and an alternate method of pain management will be needed. Motor block-stop or reduce the infusion.

Confusion Related to Opioid Use—Reduce or stop the infusion and ask for a trial of an LA infusion only to reduce the effect of the opioid.

Hypotension Related to Local Anesthetic Use Causing Vasodilatation Resulting in Periods of Hypotension—Boluses with IV fluids may be needed to maintain adequate blood pressure.

For specific medications and interventions, see the epidural order set, Figure 13.3.

Treating Side Effects and Special Considerations

Sedation/Oversedation

As with all forms of opioids, oversedation with ensuing respiratory depression is a possibility. The overall rates of respiratory depression with epidural analgesia are 0.1% to 0.9% (de Leon-Casasola, Parker, Lema, Groth, & Orsini-Fuentes, 1994). Hyrodrophilic medications, such as morphine, are thought to have the potential for delayed respiratory depression, whereas lipophilic medications, such as fentanyl, are believed to have more potential for early respiratory depression (Hurley et al., 2010). The use of supplemental oxygen can skew the mechanical reading of oxygenation provided by oxygen monitoring. For a more accurate reading of blood oxygen levels, the use of capnography or end-tidal carbon dioxide monitoring is recommended. Patients with epidural analgesia will need consistent and frequent monitoring for the onset of respiratory depression.

Nausea/Vomiting

Nausea and vomiting are common side effects of opioid use. The occurrence is estimated to be between 45% and 80% of all patients (White et al., 1992). Using antiemetics, such as metoclopramide

Standard Epidural Analgesia Orders

ALLERGIES ➤	

I HEREBY AUTHORIZE THE PHARMACY TO DISPENSE A GENERIC EQUIVALENT UNLESS THE PARTICULAR DRUG IS CIRCLED.

PATIENT PLATE

STANDARD EPIDURAL ANALGESIA ORDERS

MODE: SINGLE/INTERMITTENT ☐ CONTINUOUS ☐ CONTINUOUS WITH PCEA ☐ PCEA ONLY ☐

DATE: ______________

DO NOT INJECT, FLUSH OR MANIPULATE EPIDURAL CATHETER OR CHANGE DRESSING.
*** EPIDURAL CATHETER PATIENTS MAY NOT RECEIVE LOW MOLECULAR WEIGHT HEPARINS.**

1. **DOSING FOR CONTINUOUS INFUSION/PCEA**

SELECT (✓)	AGENT/SOLUTION	INFUSION RATE	BOLUS PCEA DOSES
	Preservative Free (PF) Morphine 0.1 mg/mL in 250 mL NS	0.5 mg (5mL) per hour and titrate to effect	Not suitable for patient bolusing.
	PF Morphine 0.1 mg/mL and Bupivacaine 0.0625% in 250 mL NS	5 mL per hour and titrate to effect	Not suitable for patient bolusing.
	PF Fentanyl 5 mcg.mL and Bupivacaine 0.0625% in 250 mL NS	5-10 mL per hour and titrate to effect	5 mL with a 15 minute lockout.
	PF Fentanyl 5 mcg.mL and Bupivacaine 0.125% in 250 mL NS	**Reserved for Knee Replacement** 5-10 mL per hour	5 mL with a 15 minute lockout.
	PF Hydromorphine 0.02 mg.mL and Bupivacaine 0.0625% in 250 mL NS	5-10 mL per hour and titrate to effect	3-5 mL with a 20 minute lockout.
	Other:		

DOSING FOR INTERMITTENT OR SINGLE INJECTION (by Anesthesia ONLY)

SELECT (✓)	AGENT	DOSE	TIME	INITIALS
	PF Morphine			
	Other:			

2. Loading dose: ____________ mL.
3. Continuous infusion rate at ________ mL/hour.
4. Patient controlled dose: _____ mL. q ______ min.
5. 4 hour lockout: _______________ mL.
6. Nasal cannula Oxygen at _________ L/min.
7. Naloxone (Narcan) 0.4 mg/mL vial at the bedside.
8. Diphenhydramine (Benadryl) ________ mg, IM q ________ h., PRN for itching x2 doses.

9. **ANTIEMETICS:**

SELECT (✓)	AGENT	DOSE	ROUTE (circle)	FREQUENCY
	Promethazine	25 mg	IM/IV	q ________ h prn
	Prochlorperazine	10 mg	IM/IV/PO	q ________ h prn
	Metoclopramide	10 mg	IM/IV	q ________ h prn
	Other:		IM/IV/PO/Rect	

10. **MONITORING PARAMETERS:**

Notify the Anesthesiologist and turn off infusion for items a-f:

a. Respiratory rate less than 8 per minute and/or O_2 sat less than 90%
b. Numbness above the nipples
c. Leg weakness or numbness
d. Sedation Score of 4 (Somnolent)
e. Seizures
f. Hypotension (Systolic BP <100)

Notify the Anesthesiologist for items g-j:

g. Severe itching or pain persists after therapy
h. Urinary retention
i. Severe constipation
j. Nausea and vomiting

11. **FOR BREAKTHROUGH PAIN GIVE:** ____
12. **DO NOT GIVE ANY OTHER OPIOIDS/SEDATIVES BEFORE CHECKING WITH THE ANESTHESIOLOGIST.**

PLEASE WRITE WITH BALLPOINT PEN	UNIT SECRETARY	DATE/TIME	RN SIGNATURE	DATE/TIME	PHYSICIAN'S SIGNATURE	DATE	TIME

PART 1 - MEDICAL RECORDS PART 2 - PHARMACY

Figure 13.3 ■ Order set exemplar. *Source:* Courtesy of Suburban Hospital–Johns Hopkins Medicine, Bethesda, MD.

(Reglan), dexamethasone (Decadron), and scopolamine patches (Transderm Scōp), can help not only to reduce the effects of the nausea and vomiting but also to increase sedation.

Pruritis

Pruritis or generalized itching is one of the most common side effects of epidural analgesia, occurring in about 60% of the patients (Hurley et al., 2010). The mechanism of pruritis with epidural opioids is not well understood. It was once thought to be caused by a histamine release, but the source is now thought to be centered in the higher cerebral centers (Hurley et al., 2010). The one fact that can be confirmed is that pruritis is not a result of a true allergic reaction. It can be treated with various medications, including hydroxyzine (Atarax), naloxone (Narcan), and nalbuphine hydrochloride (Nubaine) at reduced doses.

Hypotension

The hypotension found with epidural analgesia is the direct result of the LA combined with postoperative hypovolemia. With the LA, the blood vessels dilate and decrease the fluid pressure within the vessel. If the patient is hypovolemic, the effect will be more pronounced. Fluid bolus and epidural rate reduction, if possible, are the recommended action for hypotension with epidural analgesia.

Motor Block

In some cases, epidural analgesia has a greater effect on motor function, and a blockade may be produced as a result of the LA. The incidence of motor block is higher with lumbar epidural placement (Hurley, Cohen & Wu, 2010), but the overall incidence is low at 2% to 3% of all patients (Hurley et al., 2010). Patients may first experience numbness along the lateral thigh, and if infusion rates are not decreased, the blockade can proceed across the thigh muscles, causing a loss of quadriceps strength. Patients who are receiving epidural analgesia with LA and PCEA especially should always be tested for quadriceps strength before trying to stand.

Urinary Retention

Urinary retention for patients with epidural catheters receiving infusions with opioids and LA is the result of detrusor muscle weakness from the LA effect on the spinal cord opioid receptors. The average estimated rate of urinary retention is felt to be about 10% to 30% (Hurley et al., 2010). Urinary catheters may be needed for the first days of epidural analgesia therapy to avoid urinary retention.

Anticoagulants and Epidurals

Most patients who are on epidural analgesia may require anticoagulation either as prophylaxis for thrombus formation or as a treatment, as in the case of patients undergoing a thoracotomy. In either case, the use of anticoagulants must be carefully monitored in the postoperative period. Recommendations for catheter placement and removal can be found in the following section to avoid the formation of an epidural hematoma.

Safety Issues With Epidural Infusions

One of the most dangerous and significant side effects with epidural analgesia is epidural hematoma. An epidural hematoma is created by bleeding into the epidural space caused by tissue damage, usually when the catheter is placed or removed. If the patient is anticoagulated, the potential for epidural hematoma formation is increased. Although infrequent, the seriousness of the hematoma formation cannot be minimized. Because the bleeding is taking place in a limited and confined area inside the spinal column, the expansion of the bleed creates a clot pressing on the spinal cord, leading to spinal cord compression. The cord compression can lead to a spinal cord injury and permanent paralysis if not detected in the early stages.

Patients with epidural hematoma complain of extremely severe back pain that progresses to loss of lower extremity function and loss of bowel and bladder control. Any patient with an epidural catheter who complains of extreme pain and is on anticoagulants should immediately be screened for epidural hematoma formation by computed tomography (CT) scan or magnetic resonance imaging (MRI).

Because of the significant consequences of an epidural hematoma, the American Society of Regional Anesthesia and Pain Medicine (ASRA, 2002) have drafted a position paper with criteria for use of anticoagulants with epidural patients.

These recommendations include the following:

Subcutaneous heparin—no contraindication for placement or catheter removal

Warfarin—international normalized ratio (INR) required to be less than 1.5 for catheter removal; no placement with elevated INR

Low-molecular-weight heparin—thrombophylaxis, placement 10–12 hours after last dose, removal either directly before daily dose or 10–12 hours after last dose; medication can be resumed 2 hours after catheter removal; treatment doses placement can occur 24 hours after last dose removal of catheter prior to treatment

Antiplatelet Medications

Ticlopidine—catheter placement after discontinuation of medication for 14 days

Clopidogrel—catheter placement after discontinuation of medication for 7 days

Fondaparinux—avoid using indwelling catheters (ASRA, 2002)

Epidural Catheter Migration

Epidural catheter migration from the epidural space through the dura into the spinal canal is relatively rare. The clinical sign that this should be considered is continued sedation of the patient, despite dose reductions. To confirm that the catheter has migrated, the catheter fluid can be aspirated and checked for the presence of glucose, which would indicate that the catheter has migrated into the CSF.

Epidural Abscess

The occurrence of epidural abscess is rare, cited as 1 in 1,930 in one study (Wang, Hauerberg, & Schmidt, 1999), and infection rates were listed as 1.1 in 100,00 in other reviews (Aromaa, Lahdensuu, & Cozanitis, 1997). The most recent recommendation by ASRA relates to careful use of aseptic technique when catheters are being placed to avoid any contamination that could allow for abscess formation (Horlocker et al., 2003). Patients who are experiencing an epidural abscess present with much the same complaints as those with epidural hematoma: severe back pain, neurologic changes, and fever. An MRI can clearly identify the site of the abscess formation. A delay in diagnosis can lead to a greater risk of permanent motor impairment (Davies et al., 2004).

Outcomes

The outcomes related to epidural analgesia are very good as compared with other techniques. In a Cochrane DARE review, epidural analgesia was superior for pain relief when compared with all other routes of postoperative pain control (Block et al., 2005). In a review article by Viscusi (2008), epidural analgesia was reported to improve analgesia, increase patient satisfaction, and improve clinical outcomes. Intrathecal analgesia for postoperative pain relief was tested in a large study of 5,969 adult patients by Gwirtz et al. (1999), and the findings indicated that within a 7-year period, with a large number of participants, patient satisfaction with the technique was very high and the occurrence of side effects and complications was very low.

As always, multimodal therapies are the best recommendation for postoperative pain management, but using epidural analgesia as the base can provide high benefits with few negatives. As practice evolves and more becomes known about the way that the body perceives postoperative pain and analgesic actions, better outcomes can be expected with these techniques.

Case Study

Sandra Jones, 62 years old, has been admitted for a total joint replacement. She has been diagnosed with osteoarthritis, and walking has become much more difficult, along with increased pain in the joints. She is quite anxious about her surgery and is seeing you for her preoperative workup. When you start to discuss the possibility of using epidural analgesia postoperatively, she becomes more upset. When you ask her why, she tells you that her daughter-in-law had an epidural for her last baby and it did not work at all. When you explain to Sandra that the epidural would provide her with the best type of pain relief and better mobility after surgery, she begins to consider using one for postoperative pain relief.

Questions to Consider

1. What additional information can you provide to Sandra to help her make a decision about using an epidural for her post-operative pain control?
   a. You can tell Sandra that the technique is safe and has been used for many years successfully.
   b. Patient education about postoperative pain management options will allow Sandra to make the best choice.
   c. Letting Sandra know that many patients who have used an epidural are very satisfied with their postoperative analgesia and they were able to breathe and move better after their surgery.
2. What other information would you provide for Sandra?

REFERENCES

American Pain Society. (2008). *Principles of analgesic use in the treatment of acute pain and cancer pain*. Glenview, IL: Author.

American Society of Anesthesiologists Task Force on Acute Pain Management (ASRA). (2004). Practice guidelines for acute pain management in the perioperative setting. *Anesthesiology, 100*(6), 1573–1581.

American Society of Regional Anesthesia and Pain Medicine. (2002). *Consensus statement: Regional anesthesia in the anticoagulated patient: Defining the risks.* doi/10.1002/bjs.5180/full.

Aromaa, U., Lahdensuu, M., & Cozanitis, D. A. (1997). Severe complications associated with epidural and spinal anaesthesias in Finland 1987–1993. A study based on patient insurance claims. *Acta Anaesthesiologica Scandinavica, 41,* 445–452.

Davies, D. P., Wold, R. M., Patel, R. J., Tran, A. J., Tokhi, R. N., Chan, T. C., & Vilke, G. M. (2004). The clinical presentation and impact of diagnostic delays on emergency department patients with spinal epidural abscess. *Journal of Emergency Medicine, 26,* 285–291.

de Leon-Casasola, O. A., Parker, B. M., Lema, M. J., Groth, R. I., & Orsini-Fuentes, J. (1994). Epidural analgesia versus intravenous patient-controlled analgesia. Differences in the postoperative course of cancer patients. *Regional Anesthesia, 19,* 307–315.

Eisenach, J. C., DuPen, S., Dubois, M., Miguel, R., & Allin, D. (1995). Epidural clonidine analgesia for intractable cancer pain. The epidural clonidine study group. *Pain, 61,* 391–399.

Forster, J. G., & Rosenberg, P. H. (2004). Small dose of clonidine mixed with low-dose ropivacaine and fentanyl for epidural analgesia after total knee arthroplasty. *British Journal of Anaesthesia, 93,* 670–677.

Horlocker, T. T., Wedel, D. J., Benzon, H., Brown, D. L., Enneking, F. K., Heit, J. A., . . . Yuan, C. S. (2003). Regional anesthesia in the anticoagulated patient: Defining the risks. *Regional Anesthesia and Pain Medicine, 28,* 172–197.

Hughes, D., Simmons, S. W., & Brown, J. (2003). Combine spinal-epidural versus epidural analgesia in labour. *Cochrane Database of Systematic Reviews, 4,* art. No. CDoo3401.

Hurley, R., Cohen, S., & Wu, C. (2010). Acute pain in adults. In S. Fishman, J. Ballantyne, & J. Rathmell (Eds.), *Bonica's management of pain* (4th ed., pp. 706–710). Philadephia, PA: Wolters Kluwer/Lippincott Williams & Wilkins.

Pain Management in Blunt Force Trauma (BTT) available through www.guideline.gov

Rockford, M., & DeRuyter, M. (2009). Perioperative epidural analgesia. In H. Smith (Ed.), *Current therapies in pain.* Philadelphia, PA: Elsevier.

Viscusi, E. (2008). Patient controlled drug delivery for acute postoperative pain management: A review of current and emerging technologies. *Regional Anesthesia and Pain Medicine, 33*(2), 146–158.

Wang, L. P., Hauerberg, J., & Schmidt, J. F. (1999). Incidence of spinal epidural abscess after epidural analgesia: A national 1-year survey. *Anesthesiology, 91,* 1928–1936.

White, M. J., Berghausen, E. J., Dumont, S. W., Tsueda, K., Schroeder, J. A., Vogel, R. L., . . . Huang, K. C. (1992). Side effects during continuous epidural infusion of morphine and fentanyl. *Canadian Journal of Anaesthesiology, 39,* 576–582.

14

Regional Techniques for Postoperative Pain Relief

RATIONALE FOR USE OF REGIONAL ANALGESIA

Because 30% to 80% of surgical patients report moderate to severe pain after surgery (Apfelbaum, Chen, Mehta, & Gan, 2003; McGrath et al., 2004), it is important to provide the highest level of postoperative analgesia possible. This means the use of multiple techniques to control pain. The use of regional anesthesia has been recommended by the American Society of Anesthesiologists (ASA, 2004) as a means of extending the superior pain management of the operating room. There are two main techniques that are used: intraoperative neural blockade, a one-time procedure, and continuous peripheral nerve or wound catheters.

By using a blockade or continuous infusion of local anesthetic, the use of opioids can be minimized in the postoperative setting, resulting in fewer adverse effects, such as nausea and vomiting. The level of pain relief with a regional analgesia technique is superior to opioids alone and reduces opioid-related side effects, such as nausea, vomiting, sedation, and pruritis (Le Wendling & Enneking, 2008; Liu & Salinas, 2003; Richman et al., 2005). Pain relief and functionality are improved with the use of peripheral catheters (PCs), and functionality has been reported as improved with PCs (Rosenquist & Rosenberg, 2003). There is also some indication that the use of regional anesthesia, epidurals, and PCs has a positive impact on mortality and morbidity with high-risk patients (Hanna, Murphy, Kumar, & Wu, 2009).

The current-day anesthesia provider has many more options for increasing the effectiveness of postoperative analgesia by extending the controlled anesthetic and analgesic techniques of the operating room into the postoperative time period. Using single injections for regional blockade and inserting a PC that can provide extended adjunct pain relief can help surgical patients or trauma patients recover faster with fewer side effects.

Intraoperative Blockade

An intraoperative blockade can be used to reduce pain in the immediate postoperative period. There are various blocks that can be used, such as plexus, ilioinguinal, penile, axillary, or femoral. The use of a blockade can extend the analgesia of the operating room into the first hours of the recovery period. The disadvantage of using a single block is the limited effect. Postoperative one-time blocks can last for up to 24 hours but tend to wear off in a relatively short period (Hurley, Cohen, & Wu, 2010). The use of epinephrine in the block solution can help extend the action of the block.

Solutions that are used for blocks are local anesthetics. Solutions that have rapid onset combined with a short duration of action include 2% lidocaine and 1.5% mepivacaine (Wallace & Staats, 2005). Solutions that have extended action but a slower onset include 0.5% bupivacaine, 0.75% ropivacaine, and 0.5% levobupivacaine (Wallace & Staats, 2005).

These single-dose intraoperative blocks can be placed in a wide variety of surgical locations. The blocks are designed to provide lack of sensation to the surgical area, and they are done with a local anesthesia, such as bupivacaine, that can have an extended action if epinephrine is included in the block solution.

Areas that are commonly used for blockade include axillary, interscalene, femoral, and sciatic.

Axillary

This block is used for upper extremity surgery, such as shoulder surgery. It is used for procedures of the forearm, wrist, and hand, chronic pain syndromes, and vascular diseases. It blocks the terminal branches of the brachial plexus.

Interscalene

This block is commonly used for open-shoulder surgery, rotator cuff repair, acromioplasty, shoulder arthroplasty, and proximal upper limb surgery (May & DeRuyter, 2009). The block performed is a brachial plexus block. When performed as a surgical adjunct, this block may not produce analgesia for the ulnar nerve, the loading bolus may produce phrenic nerve block, and the patient can develop hoarseness from laryngeal blockade, as well as Horner's syndrome as a result of sympathetic blockade.

Femoral

The femoral block is commonly used for surgeries of the knee and femur. Analgesia for the anterior thigh, femur, and most of the knee joint is produced with blockade. It can be combined with a sciatic block, which effectively blocks both the anterior and posterior aspects of the knee. These blocks have been most effective when a continuous local anesthetic infusion is used, leading to improved patient outcomes and side effects in the postoperative period. Careful assessment is needed to determine if there is muscle weakness in the lower extremity, primarily quadriceps muscle weakness, with the block before getting the patient out of bed to avoid buckling of the extremity. Some of the more important patient outcomes when this block is used are increased ability to move the surgical joint, opioid sparing, decreased side effects such as postoperative nausea and vomiting (PONV), and increased patient satisfaction.

Sciatic

Sciatic blocks provide anesthesia to the skin of the posterior thigh, hamstring, biceps muscle, and part of the hip and knee joint, and the entire leg below the knee with the exception of the skin of the lower leg. It can be combined with a femoral block for knee surgery or lumbar plexus block for hip and femur surgery.

Thoracic Paravertebral

The thoracic paravertebral block is commonly used for surgeries of the breast and chest wall, and for abdominal surgeries. Other uses for this type of block include anesthesia and/or analgesia for herniorrhaphy, iliac crest bone grafts, soft tissue mass excisions, and analgesic adjunct for laparoscopic surgery, cholecystectomy, nephrectomy, appendectomy, thorocotomy, obstetric analgesia, minimally invasive cardiac surgery, and hip surgery. Positive patient outcomes with this type of block include reduction in pain scores, opioid-sparing effect, decreased PONV, and decreased length of stay (May & DeRuyter, 2009; Melton & Liu, 2010; Wallace & Staats, 2005).

Peripheral Catheters for Postoperative Analgesia

In certain patient populations, such as orthopedic total joint replacement patients, where high levels of pain are expected, using pain medications in conjunction with a PC infusion has become the accepted practice. The prior practice pattern for these orthopedic patients was to use epidural catheters for postoperative analgesia. The change in practice was partially stimulated by the focus on prophylactic anticoagulation in these patients and the recognition of increased potential for adverse effects such as epidural hematoma. The American Society for Regional Anesthesia (ASRA, 2002) developed a consensus statement related to anesthesiologist practice with epidural catheters and anticoagulation, which outlines recommendations for practice when epidural catheters are used for postoperative pain relief in patients receiving anticoagulants. As a result of this paper and the recognition of the increased risk of epidural hematoma with the use of epidurals and anticoagulants, the use of epidural catheters with orthopedic patients decreased dramatically over a year or two.

This decrease in epidural use made way for the development of alternate methods of pain control for total joint replacement patients using a combined medication and regional analgesia technique with PC. Because multimodal analgesia is always recommended as the best approach to postoperative pain management (ASA, 2004), this new technique is a good addition to the options that surgeons and anesthesia providers are able to offer patients.

The PC is similar to an epidural catheter that can be placed by the surgeon in or near an incision to provide localized pain relief, or the PC can be placed by an anesthesiologist along a nerve, such as the femoral nerve, sciatic nerve, or both, for patients with knee surgery or interscalene brachial plexus to provide continuous pain relief for shoulder or arm surgery. With either type of placement, the patient can expect to have the catheter remain in place while infusions of local anesthetic, such as bupivacaine or ropivacaine, infuse through the catheter.

Most PCs use some type of infusion device to provide continuous flow. One example is the ON-Q pump (Figure 14.1), an elastomeric device that can be configured to deliver a preset rate continuous flow, or as a variable flow rate, or the patient can self-administer a bolus dose. During or before surgery, the catheter is inserted into the area where blockade is desired. A ball-shaped reservoir is filled with a local anesthetic solution. The ON-Q infusion is complete in several days, when the ball containing the medication collapses and is no longer firm to touch. There are various infusion devices available that work in basically the same fashion and each has its own advantages and disadvantages. The additional option of a patient-controlled button device can allow the patient to provide a bolus dose of local anesthetic when needed.

Placement of Peripheral Catheter

To place a peripheral nerve catheter, the anesthesia provider uses a hollow Touhy-type needle connected to a nerve stimulator or an ultrasound. Once placement has been confirmed, the provider threads

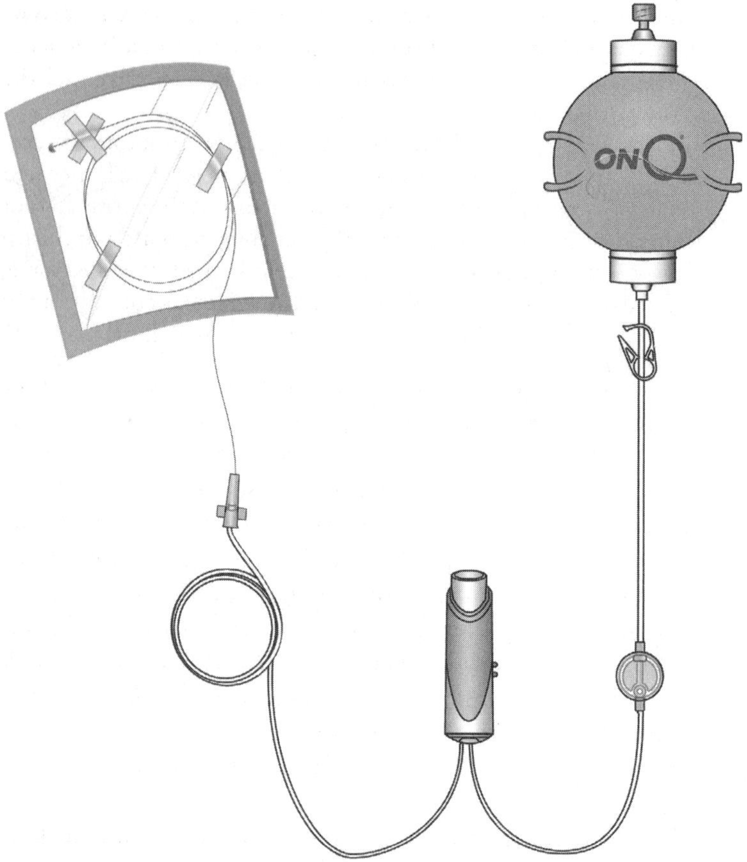

Figure 14.1 ■ ON-Q pump. *Source:* Used by permission of I-Flow Corp.

the catheter down the hollow center of the needle to the area that needs analgesia. To test placement, the provider confirms location with one of two techniques.

1. Nerve stimulator (NS): To locate the correct site for placement using an NS, the anesthesia provider uses a short, beveled Teflon-coated needle inserted into the area for blockade attached to an NS with a

pulse duration of 0.15 milliseconds. The correct nerves are located by the twitches elicited by the stimulation. The stimulation intensity is reduced after the block is injected, the catheter is inserted, and the needle is removed.

2. Ultrasound (US)-guided peripheral nerve block: To locate the correct site for placement with ultrasound, a short, beveled Teflon-coated needle is inserted into the area for blockade so that the entire shaft of the needle is in the ultrasound beam, and both the shaft and the tip of the needle are visualized. Once the site is located, the injection is completed and the catheter is threaded through the needle. Spread of local anesthetic is confirmed with continuous sonography.

The onset of blockade with US has been reported as faster compared with the older nerve stimulation technique. There is Level 1b evidence to make a grade A recommendation for the use of ultrasound. This technique improves onset and success of sensory blockade, decreased local anesthetic needs, and decreased time to perform lower extremity blockade (Salinas, 2010). Indications not entirely favorable to the use of ultrasound include the same effects noted for tissue damage to neighboring structures and inadequate analgesia in a small number of patients (Casati et al., 2009; LeWendling & Enneking, 2008). Nerves that can be blocked using continuous local anesthetic infusion for continued analgesia after surgery include those that were described earlier in the chapter for block locations.

The risks of using a PC are very low. Nerve injury with blocks is estimated to be from 0% to 10% with upper extremity single shot blocks and 0.5% with lower extremity blocks (Melton & Liu, 2010). Systemic local anesthetic toxicity is reported as rare (Bleckner et al., 2010). Pneumothorax rates are reported as low with both interscalene and paravertebral blocks. Infections with blocks and catheters are rare (Capdevila, Bringuier, & Borgeat, 2009). ASRA has recommended the use of aseptic technique for catheter placements with monitoring of infections.

The use of local anesthetic catheters has moved into new areas and found acceptance in the popular press. In 2006, *The New York Times* reported on an anesthesiologist who recognized the positive benefits of using local anesthetic infusions to help relieve battle wounds in the leg and arm (McGough, 2006). He used a small compact infusion pump with local anesthetic as adjunct pain relief for soldiers in military hospitals. This technique allowed for immediate decreases in pain and helping to continue pain relief as the soldiers were transported to other military facilities for surgery or rehabilitation.

A PC should always have a secondary method of pain relief, such as PCA or intermittent IV analgesic, in case of PC failure or dislodgement. The value of using a PC is related to the use of two different types of analgesia—multimodal analgesia using local anesthetic in the pump and intravenous opioids, an opioid-sparing effect, and a reduction in side effects such as nausea. Increases in patient satisfaction, although difficult to determine, have been reported with the use of PCs as in decreased length of stay. Meta-analyses have shown a reduction of 1 day of hospitalization (Liu, Richman, Thirlby, & Wu, 2006). Technical failure is rare (1%), as is local anesthetic toxicity (0%), and wound infection rates are below control group rates (0.7%) (Liu et al., 2006). Given that the cost of the pump is low, ranging from $200 to $280 per patient (Ilfeld, Morey, & Enneking, 2004), and the outcomes are very good, this economical local anesthetic infusion option provides added benefit for patients, health care providers, and hospitals and has dramatically improved postoperative pain management.

Case Study

Steven Jones, 72 years old, has been diagnosed with lung cancer and is being admitted for a thoracotomy for the removal of part of his left lung. The surgeon explains that he will remove as much of the lung cancer as he can and do biopsies to check for any spread of the disease. Steven is concerned about having a surgery that is in his chest. He feels that it will be very painful, and he has had trouble with unrelieved pain with past surgeries, which were not as difficult. The surgeon defers to the anesthesia provider to help Steven make his decision about how to manage Steven's pain in the postoperative period. Steven has mild hypertension and congestive heart disease. He takes a daily low-dose aspirin. If you were the anesthesia provider, what kind of information could you provide to Steven?

Questions to Consider

1. Because thoracotomy is one of the surgeries for high level of pain, what combination of analgesic techniques would provide the best type of pain relief?
2. Would the anticoagulation provided by the low-dose aspirin affect the choice of epidural anesthesia or peripheral catheter postoperatively?
3. Will the use of intraoperative blockade or PC make any difference in the outcome of Steven's surgery?
4. Could you combine an epidural catheter with a PC?

REFERENCES

American Society of Anesthesiologists. (2004). *Practice guidelines for acute pain management in the perioperative setting.* Park Ridge, IL: Author.

American Society of Regional Anesthesia and Pain Management. (2002). *Consensus statement: Regional anesthesia in the anticoagulated patient: Defining the risks.* doi/10.1002/bjs.5180/full.

Apfelbaum, J. L., Chen, C., Mehta, S. S., & Gan, T. J. (2003). Postoperative pain experience: Results form a national survey suggest postoperative pain continues to be undermanaged. *Anesthesia and Analgesia*, *97*, 534–540.

Bleckner, L. L., Bina, S., Kwon, K. H., McKnight, G., Dragovich, A., & Buckenmaier, C., III. (2010). Serum ropivacaine concentrations and systemic local anesthetic toxicity in trauma patients receiving long-term continuous peripheral nerve block catheters. *Anesthesia and Analgesia*, *110*(2), 630–634.

Capdevila, X., Bringuier. S., & Borgeat, A. (2009). Infectious risk of continuous peripheral nerve blocks. *Anesthesiology*, *100*, 182–188.

Casati, A., Danelli, G., Baciarello, M., Corradi, M., Leone, S., Di Cianni, S., & Fanelli, G. (2009). A prospective, randomized comparison between ultrasound and nerve stimulation guidance for multiple injection axillary brachial plexus block. *Survey of Anesthesiology*, *53*(4), 186–189.

Hanna, M., Murphy, J., Kumar, K., & Wu, C. (2009). Regional techniques and outcome: What is the evidence? *Current Opinion in Anaesthesiology*, *22*, 672–677.

Ilfeld, B. M., Le, L. T., Ramjohn, J., Loland, V. J., Wadhwa, A. N., Gerancher, J. C., . . . Horlocker, T. T. (2009). The effects of local anesthetic concentration and dose on continuous infraclavicular nerve blocks: A multicenter, randomized, observer-masked, controlled study. *Anesthesia and Analgesia*, *108*(1), 345–350.

Le-Wendling, L., & Enneking, F. K. (2008). Continuous peripheral nerve blockade for postoperative analgesia. *Current Opinion in Anaesthesiology*, *21*, 602–609.

Liu, S. S., Richman, J. M., Thirlby, R. C., & Wu, C. L. (2006). Efficacy of continuous wound catheters delivering local anesthetic for postoperative analgesia: A quantitative and qualitative systematic review of randomized controlled trials. *Journal of the American College of Surgeons*, *203*(6), 914–932.

Liu, S. S., & Salinas, F. V. (2003). Continuous plexus and peripheral nerve blocks for postoperative analgesia. *Anesthesia and Analgesia*, *96*(1), 263–272.

May, E., & Deruyter, M. (2009). Continuous peripheral nerve catheter techniques. In H. Smith (Ed.), *Current therapy in pain* (pp. 84–92). Philadelphia, PA: Elsevier.

McGough, R. (2006). Pain pump tested in battle. *The Wall Street Journal*.

McGrath, B., Elgendy, H., Chung, F., Kamming, D., Curti, B., & King, S. (2004). Thirty percent of patients have moderate to severe pain 24 hr after ambulatory surgery: A survey of 5,703 patients. *Canadian Journal of Anesthesia*, *51*, 886–891.

Melton, S., & Liu, S. (2010). Chapter 52. In S. Fishman, J. Ballantyne, & J. Rathmell (Eds.), *Bonica's management of pain* (5th ed.). Philadelphia, PA: Lippincott Williams & Wilkins.

Richman, J. M., Liu, S. S., Courpas, G., Wong, R., Rowlingson, A. J., McGready, J., . . . Wu, C. L. (2006). Does continuous peripheral nerve block provide superior pain control to opioids? A meta-analysis. *Anesthesia and Analgesia*, *102*(1), 248–257.

Rosenquist, R., & Rosenberg, J. (2003). Postoperative pain guidelines. *Regional Anesthesia*, *28*(4), 279–288.

Salinas, F. V. (2010). Ultrasound and review of evidence for lower extremity peripheral nerve blocks. *Regional Anesthesia and Pain Medicine*, *35*(2, Suppl. 1), S16–S25.

Wallace, M., & Staats, P. (2005). *Pain medicine and management: Just the facts*. New York, NY: McGraw-Hill.

V

Difficult-to-Treat Patient Populations

15

Chronic Pain Patients With Acute Pain

THE PATIENT WITH CHRONIC AND ACUTE PAIN

The patient with chronic and acute pain is one of the most difficult to treat and time-consuming patients when seen in the clinic or admitted to the hospital. The patient may be having surgery, be seen after injury or trauma, or be admitted for treatment of uncontrolled pain. No matter what the cause, the situation can be stressful for the patient, the health care provider, and the nursing staff.

The reasons the situation can be stressful include a combination of many factors.

- The patient may have had previous experiences with the health care system that were not positive.
- Health care providers may see opioid-dependent patients who have chronic pain as "drug seeking" or falsely label them as "addicted."
- The patient's report of pain may not be accepted as real and the patient may, in turn, be forced to validate or prove that the pain he or she is experiencing is real.
- The patient's expectations may be that increased medication is the answer, when in fact, other types of therapy or treatments may be more beneficial.
- Health care providers may be reluctant to restart high-dose opioids after surgery or trauma, making it more difficult to control the new pain (D'Arcy, 2010).

Chronic, now called persistent, pain accounts for 40 million patient visits annually and is the most common reason that patients seek help for pain from their health care providers. On average, the patient with chronic pain presents with the following:

- Has had pain for 7 years
- Has had three major surgeries
- Has incurred medical bills of $50,000 to $100,000 (Pain Advocacy Community, 2004)

There are many different types of chronic pain. According to a survey by Research America, the most common types of chronic pain include back pain (28%), arthritis and joint pain (19%), headaches and migraines (17%), knee pain (17%), and shoulder pain (7%). Although it is difficult to measure precisely, chronic pain costs an estimated $100 billion per year related to health care costs, welfare and disability costs, losses in tax revenue, and lost productivity through both absenteeism and presenteeism. The worker who comes to work but is in pain (presenteeism) can be just as costly as the worker who does not come to work (absenteeism).

Because chronic pain is so prevalent, it is inevitable that health care providers will be seeing numerous patients with chronic pain conditions who also have an acute pain complaint. There are only about 6,000 pain specialists in practice nationally, so access to pain management professionals is very limited, and appointment times for chronic pain clinics can require months of waiting. Because the health care provider will need to treat these patients, it is important for the health care provider to know how to assess and select appropriate treatment options.

One of the biggest drawbacks to treating an opioid-tolerant patient with chronic pain when he or she presents with acute pain is the need to prescribe additional opioids for the new pain. In a survey with 400 nurse practitioners, the respondents indicated that the number two and three barriers to prescribing opioids were fear of addicting the patients to the medication and fear of regulatory oversight of their prescribing practice with opioids (D'Arcy, 2009). These responses indicate that there is a concern on the part of the health care providers prescribing the opioids that may color their practice when having to escalate opioid doses. Because patients with chronic pain need higher medication doses to control their pain, the medication requirements for managing the new acute pain will be higher than the medication requirements for the patient with the same injury who is not taking daily opioids.

There can be a misunderstanding about the use of the current medications to treat both the chronic and the new pain. When patients with chronic pain are injured or have surgery, some health care providers have the misconception that the medications used to treat the chronic pain will be sufficient to treat the additional surgical pain. This misunderstanding will lead to significantly undertreated pain in the postoperative period. This may create an adversarial relationship between the health care provider and the patient and result in behaviors such as angry outbursts or reluctance to change medications that would not be the usual response to the situation.

Clinical Pearl

Medication dosages based on an opioid-naïve patient's medication needs will not be sufficient to relieve acute pain in patients who regularly take large opioid doses to manage daily chronic pain.

No matter what the cause of the acute pain, the patient with chronic pain can create a situation in which there is conflict over medications and pain management and resistance to the proposed plan of care. Understanding the needs of patients with chronic pain when they are admitted to the acute care setting or come to an outpatient clinic with a new or different pain complaint can make treating patients less difficult and provide better pain relief for patients.

DIFFERENCES IN ACUTE AND CHRONIC PAIN

There are distinct differences in acute and chronic pain.

- *Acute pain* is the result of trauma or injury. It serves the purpose of alerting the body that an injury or tissue damage has occurred (American Pain Society [APS], 2006, 2008). It can create anxiety, fear, diaphoresis, pallor, and changes in vital signs such as blood pressure and heart rate. The patient expects acute pain to be short in duration, and a full recovery is anticipated.
- *Chronic pain*, on the other hand, serves no purpose. Chronic or persistent pain is pain that lasts beyond the normal healing period (APS, 2006, 2008). Patients with chronic pain can be anxious, but most often they are depressed. The suicide rate for patients with chronic pain is twice the national average (Tang & Crane, 2006). The patient with chronic pain has physiologic changes that make the pain more intense and the response to pain medications decreased. In some cases, chronic pain can be the result of undertreated or untreated acute pain (e.g., complex regional pain syndrome [CRPS]) in which the pain becomes a self-perpetuating entity and no new pain stimulus is required for the pain to continue.

To further complicate the concept of pain differentiation, chronic pain can have various sources, such as musculoskeletal, visceral, somatic, or neuropathic. Most health care providers understand the idea of musculoskeletal or visceral pain, but neuropathic pain may mean the condition is much harder to assess, diagnose, and treat.

Neuropathic Pain

Neuropathic pain is a type of chronic pain that results from the injury of the nerves of the peripheral or central nervous system. One of the newest definitions of neuropathic pain is pain arising as a direct consequence of a lesion or disease of the somatosensory system (Treede et al., 2008). Neuropathic pain is resistant to many commonly used treatments for pain relief. In a study of randomized trials, only one half of the patients experienced even partial pain relief (Dworkin et al., 2010). This means that the patient with a new acute pain and a neuropathic pain condition will present with pain only partially relieved at best.

Physiologic Changes With Chronic Pain

The patient with chronic pain comes to the experience of acute pain with an altered physiology. Especially with neuropathic pain, the neural pathways become sensitized to pain, and the neurons change their patterns and pain processing. This effect is called *neuronal plasticity*. This can produce a phenomenon called *wind-up* in which a small pain stimulus can elicit a very high-intensity pain. This is an important fact for health care providers to know and understand when they are discussing pain with the patient. Patients with chronic pain will have continuous high-intensity pain related to the changes in their physiology and the lessened effect of pain medications. This is not something the patient can control; it is a natural effect of chronic persistent pain.

Other changes that take place in the patient's facilitating and inhibiting pain mediators include the following:

- Pain-facilitating substances, such as substance P, are secreted from peripheral nerve endings with production of tumor necrosis factor and kinins such as bradykinin.
- Neural pathways become sensitized and *N*-methyl-d-aspartate (NMDA) receptors are activated to process the pain quicker and with more intensity (Dubner, 2005).
- The patient's immune response is diminished because natural killer cells, those cells programmed to kill tumor or virus-infected cells, are suppressed.

Thus, it is no wonder that patients with chronic pain and a new acute pain do not appear the same as those patients with similar complaints but no chronic pain. To recognize these patients when taking the history and physical, it is a good idea to take a full pain history from the patients.

THE HISTORY AND PHYSICAL

It is important to recognize the patient with chronic pain as early as possible in the treatment or hospitalization. Aside from the usual questions that are asked by the health care provider, it is important to ask about any pain conditions that the patient currently has. Red flags should go up with any of the following conditions:

- Fibromyalgia
- Osteoarthritis or rheumatoid arthritis
- Chronic pain from low back pain, spinal stenosis, whiplash, or any musculoskeletal injury
- Neuropathic pain syndromes, such as painful diabetic neuropathy, postherpetic neuralgia, postmastectomy pain syndrome, postthoracotomy pain syndrome, or CRPS
- Cyclical pain syndromes, such as sickle-cell disease or migraine headaches
- Failed back syndrome or degenerative disc disease
- Repeated surgical procedures
- Chronic infection, such as osteomyelitis

Once one of these conditions have been identified, it is a signal that this patient will need special attention to pain management and further discussion is needed. The health care provider should also listen to the way the patient describes the pain because verbal descriptors can often give clues as to the source of the pain. Pain can be either nociceptive or neuropathic.

Examples of nociceptive and neuropathic pain verbal descriptors are the following:

- Nociceptive pain, which can be visceral or somatic—descriptors such as constant, achy, visceral cramping, or sharp
- Neuropathic pain—descriptors such as burning, shooting, sharp, painful, numbness, pain that resembles an electric shock, painful itching, or a complaint of strange sensations (APS, 2006)

The health care provider will also need to discuss what treatment works best for the patient's pain and which medications are most effective. In many cases, the patient may have seen as many as five or six health care providers and tried multiple medications and doses, so relying on the patient to guide medication choices is one way to ensure that the patient will have a good chance of adequate pain relief.

It is also imperative to get correct medication doses. The health care provider who can retrieve this information from the electronic medical record has an advantage. Some patients who have had a bad experience when hospitalized may increase their usual medication doses when giving the history to ensure that they will have adequate pain relief when they have surgery. If medication doses are inflated, this creates a patient safety issue because it is possible to oversedate an opioid-dependent patient if enough opioid is provided. The health care provider should make all efforts to confirm the correct medication doses, and if electronic confirmation is not possible, contacting the prescribing practitioner may be necessary. As always, the final decision on medication is the health care provider's, but listening to the patient will avoid mistakes that past health care providers have made.

For opioid-dependent patients having surgery, make sure that they take their usual morning dose of medication prior to arriving at the hospital. Missing doses of medication in the preoperative period will set the patient back, decrease medication blood levels, and create a situation in the postanesthesia care unit (PACU) in which the patient must catch up with the missed medication as well as treat the new surgical pain. Once the procedure is completed, restarting the opioid medication as soon as possible once the patient can tolerate fluids will help control the pain more effectively in the immediate postoperative period.

Assessing pain in this type of patient will require more than just a simple 0–10 rating scale. It can be very discouraging to hear of an 8/10 pain intensity despite trials of various medications and techniques. Using the numeric rating scale (NRS) will most often result in continued high pain ratings. Many patients with chronic pain have daily pain scores that are midrange (5–6/10). Asking the patient about his or her best daily pain rating will give the health care provider a goal pain rating. Additionally, it is important to ask the patient what his or her pain level is with activity and at rest. This will provide the health care provider with an idea of what will be needed for physical therapy or postoperative activity. If the pain regimen can reduce the current pain to a level close to the best daily pain rating, the patients will be able to function at preadmission or preinjury functional levels. Using an interview-structured pain assessment tool, such as the Brief Pain Impact Questionnaire (BPIQ), will provide a structured method of obtaining all the salient information related to the patient's pain complaint and past pain history (see Chapter 4 for information on the BPIQ).

Clinical Pearl

If the patient with low back pain complains of a constant pain that worsens at night and cannot be relieved with medication, position changes, or other pain relief techniques, consider that the pain may be malignant in origin and provide a complete workup to rule out a malignant source.

THE PLAN OF CARE

The plan of care for a patient who has chronic as well as acute pain is not as simple as just increasing opioid medications. There are several key concepts that will need to be addressed so that the pain can be effectively managed.

- Develop a trusting and nonjudgmental relationship. If the patient feels you believe his or her report of pain and will act in good faith to relieve the pain, he or she will be more open and a positive outcome can be achieved.
- Set realistic and achievable goals. Being pain free is not a goal that can be reached with a patient who has chronic pain. Ask the patient about his or her daily pain levels and set a goal that can be reached.
- Use various medications and techniques to relieve the pain. Adding in regional analgesia, behavioral techniques, and rehabilitation approaches will offer the patient the best chance to meet his or her goals.

- For the outpatient, determine who will be the primary prescriber. This person should be the one who writes all prescriptions for pain management.
- If the patient is seeing a pain management specialist, the patient may have a signed agreement about opioid prescribing. The health care provider seeing the patient for the new injury or surgery should contact this prescriber to tell him or her about any new medication needs.

One important concept that needs to be addressed for this category of patients is the need for higher doses of pain medication. They will need additional medication to control the acute pain until healing occurs. For surgical patients who are highly opioid dependent, they may need a continuous infusion on a patient-controlled analgesia and frequent breakthrough medications to control pain from therapy or activity. The health care provider should make it clear that this is just a temporary increase and that the patient should be able to return to his or her baseline medications once healing occurs.

Each patient with chronic pain who presents with an acute pain condition is an individual. There is no clear-cut rule as to how to manage these patients. Their needs are complex, and care can be time consuming. Using clear communication and creating a nonjudgmental climate for interactions can provide the base on which to build a therapeutic relationship with the patient.

Case Study

John P. has had four surgeries to repair the damage to his back after a motor vehicle accident. With each surgery, he is optimistic but has had poor results to date. He rates his daily pain at 6/10 and it can increase to 10/10 if he needs to move quickly, walk stairs, or stay on his feet for a long period. He can care for himself but has had to file for disability because he cannot sit for any length of time, stand for a long period, or lift or carry heavy items. Unfortunately, because of his unstable gait, John has fallen and has a femur fracture. He needs surgical repair but is anxious about pain control. He has had some very negative experiences with the health care system as a whole in the past. His current pain management regimen is methadone 10 mg, 4 times per day, with a morphine immediate release (MSIR) of 10 to 20 mg every 4 hours for breakthrough pain. You are assigned to manage John's pain in the postoperative period. What kinds of issues will come into play?

Questions to Consider

1. As you are taking the history and physical, you realize that John has long-standing chronic pain with opioid dependency. How will this affect your plan of care?
2. What is the best method of assessing pain in John's case?
3. John is using methadone as a long-acting medication, how will you compensate for the medication when he is taking nothing by mouth for surgery and in the immediate postoperative period?
4. What can you tell John that will make him feel that you are concerned about his pain relief and will make all honest efforts to manage his pain?
5. Should you be concerned about addicting John to the medication in this period or fear that your prescribing pattern will be questioned?

REFERENCES

American Pain Society. (2006). *Pain control in the primary care setting.* Glenview, IL: Author.

American Pain Society. (2008). *Principles of analgesic use in the treatment of acute pain and cancer pain*. Glenview, IL: Author.

D'Arcy, Y. (2009). Be in the know about pain management. *The Nurse Practitioner, 34*(4), 43–47.

D'Arcy, Y. (2010). Managing chronic pain in acute care: Getting it right. *Nursing 2010, 40*(4), 48–51.

Dubner, R. (2005). Plasticity in central nociceptive pathways. In H. Merskey, J. D. Loeser, & R. Dubner (Eds.), *The paths of pain, 1975–2005.* Seattle, WA: The International Association for the Study of Pain Press.

Dworkin, R. H., O'Connor, A. B., Audette, J., Baron, R., Gourlay, G., Haanpää, M. L., . . . Wells, C. D. (2010). Recommendations for the pharmacological management of neuropathic pain: An overview and literature update. *Mayo Clinic Proceedings, 85*(Suppl. 3), S3–S14.

Pain Advocacy Community. (2004). Available at www.partnersagainstpain .com/pain advocacy

Tang, N. K., & Crane, C. (2006). Suicidality in chronic pain: A review of the prevalence, risk factors, and psychological links. *Psychological Medicine, 36*(5), 575–586.

Treede, R. D., Jensen, T. S., Campbell, J. N., Cruccu, G., Dostrovsky, J. O., Griffin, J. W., . . . Serra, J. (2008). Neuropathic pain: Redefinition and a grading system for clinical research purposes. *Neurology, 70*(18), 1630–1635.

16

Sickle Disease

SICKLE-CELL DISEASE

Sickle-cell anemia was known in Africa before the 20th century by many different names. It was formally identified in 1920 by a Chicago physician who treated a Black student from the West Indies (Ballas, 2010). It was not until the mid-1900s that the disease was determined to be a molecular disease that presented with abnormal red blood cells that were sickle shaped (Ballas, 2010). Sickle-cell disease is a collection of genetic blood disorders that includes sickle-cell anemia. The focus of treatment for this condition is to control symptoms such as pain and infections.

Historically, there was value in having only one sickle-cell gene called the sickle-cell trait. In the areas of the world where this disease was common, having the sickle-cell trait was protection from malaria. The disease is found not only in people with African American heritage but also in people of Native American, East Indian, Greek, Italian, Eastern Asian, and Hispanic descent (Brookoff, 2009).

Today, sickle-cell anemia has been determined to be one of the most common hereditary hematologic disorders associated with periods of latency and high activity. It affects approximately 70,000 Americans (Gevirtz, 2008) whose crises can range from less than one per year to as frequently as on an annual basis. During periods of activity, the patient with sickle-cell disease will come into a clinic or hospital emergency department (ED) in a vaso-occlusive crisis complaining of severe pain, which is the main reason that patients seek help from health care providers. During periods of latency the patient may have no pain or only mild pain and be able to maintain a normal lifestyle.

This condition is cyclic in nature. Patients may do well for months and then require a hospitalization for pain management. The crises can be sparked by any number of causes, such as changes in temperature or dehydration. The health care provider who has to treat patients with sickle-cell disease will need to know not only how to manage the patient when the disease is not active but also how to control the severe pain when it occurs.

Pathophysiology

Because many of the patients with sickle-cell disease have been through multiple crises, there is a varying amount of damage at the cellular level. Some patients will have early entries into their medical records of strokes as young children when the occlusion of the vessels occurred in the cerebral tissue.

To confirm a diagnosis of sickle-cell disease, the patient must have at least one sickle-cell gene in which hemoglobin-S makes up at least one half of the hemoglobin (Gevirtz, 2008). Vaso-occlusion is the hallmark clinical occurrence (Ballas, 2007, 2010; Buchanan, Woodward, & Reed, 2005; Elliot & Simpson, 2010; Gevirtz, 2008). This crisis is identified by severe pain from narrowing and occlusion of microvasculature and, at times, macrovasculature (Ballas, 2007). There are several stages to cause the sickling of the red blood cells that results in vaso-occlusion.

1. Red blood cells are damaged by repeated deoxygenating cycles, eventually leading to the creation of sickle-shaped red blood cells. Other processes that promote cell deformity include dehydration, acidosis, and temperature changes.
2. Chronic inflammation can result from repeated polymerization, allowing the deformed cells to easily adhere to the vascular endothelium. This process occurs with a multitude of inflammatory mediators, such as bradykinin, cytokines, and prostaglandins, resulting in chronic

vascular inflammation (Ballas, 2007; Brookoff, 2009; Gevirtz, 2008; Platt, Beasley, Miller, & Eckman, 2002).

The end result of this sickling process creates a multitude of conditions that affect the patient's overall health status, such as the following:

- Anemia
- Vaso-occlusive crisis in which small capillaries and vessels become blocked leading to painful infarcts in bone or potentially cerebral vascular accidents
- Damage to major organs, such as spleen, liver, kidneys, and lungs
- Increased susceptibility to infections
- Acute chest syndrome
- Multiorgan dysfunction syndrome resulting in mental status changes, rhabdomyolysis with myalgia, darkened urine, and extreme pain
- Dactylitis (hand–foot syndrome) in younger patients as the result of infarcts in bones
- Priapism
- Cholecystitis from increased turnover of hemoglobin
- Acute headache as a precursor of cerebral infarct (Anie & Green, 2009; Brookoff, 2009; Gevirtz, 2008; Platt et al., 2002)

No matter what the result of the sickling process, each of the conditions can produce severe and excruciating pain. For younger patients, the continued pain seems to be uncontrollable, and the unknown frequency with which it occurs can produce profound anxiety. Family members who are carriers of the sickle-cell trait may feel guilty at having passed along such a painful condition to their child. Guilt may also affect those family members who do not have the active disease but must witness a brother or sister going through the pain.

Diagnosing the Patient Who Is in Sickle-Cell Crisis

Pain is the primary complaint when a sickle-cell crisis is occurring. As the patient progresses through the crisis, other conditions occur, such as the following:

- Increased pain associated with anxiety and anorexia
- Decreased hemoglobin with an increase in the percentage of dense red blood cells

- Increased red cell distribution width and increased hemoglobin distribution width
- Continued severe level pain with fevers, joint swelling, and effusions
- Anemia, reticulocytosis, leukocytosis, increases in C-reactive protein and fibrinogen, lactate dehydrogenase, and creatine phosphokinase

As the crisis resolves, the pain levels decrease and laboratory values gradually return to baseline.

Assessing the Patient With Sickle-Cell Disease

Patients with sickle-cell disease have periods when their pain can be well controlled with a mild analgesic, such as acetaminophen or a nonsteroidal anti-inflammatory drug (NSAID). At other times, they are dependent on intravenous (IV) opioids to control the pain of crisis. The health care provider will see patients through all of these varied presentations and will need to understand how to assess the pain associated with crisis. Many of the patients will be children or young adults who do not have the skills to deal with pain.

Using the numeric rating scale (NRS) can help determine the intensity of pain and measure the effectiveness of the pain medications for older patients. For younger patients, the FACES scale can help assess the pain.

Other key elements for assessing pain in a patient with sickle-cell disease are the following:

- Ask the patient what he or she was feeling like before the pain began and look for indicators such as increased weakness or lethargy, both indicative of anemia.
- Ask the patient if this pain is similar to the pain he or she usually has with a crisis.
- Ask the patient if he or she tried to control the pain and when he or she knew that help from a health care provider was needed.
- Assess the patient for any signs of chest syndrome, such as increased secretions, cough, fever, abnormal lung sounds, or feelings of being short of breath.
- Try to have the patient locate all the sites of pain—legs, back, chest, and so forth—to determine the extent of the sickling.

- Consider the functionality of the patient and consider what the source of any disparity could be.
- Reassess the patient frequently for any changes in pain intensity (American Pain Society [APS], 1999; Platt et al., 2002).

Most patients who have regular sickle-cell crises know what they feel like just before a crisis and can tell you that this pain is the same as they always have. Many patients will say that the bone pain is extremely painful. When infarcts are taking place in bones, the pain can be punishing.

Medications for Treating Sickle-Cell Crisis

Most patients with recurring sickle-cell crisis have been exposed to opioids as young children. They view these medications as a source of pain relief, and it is no wonder that they come to expect these medications for their pain and see these drugs as their best hope for pain relief. This does not make them all addicts; it just provides evidence of the expectations the health care system has created in these patients.

Most of the patients who are in a crisis have tried their usual pain management regimen at home, and when it proved inadequate, they come into the hospital through the ED. This means that these patients will have medical records that show repeated treatment and admissions for pain control with opioids. This does not make these patients drug seeking, but rather, self-aware of when they need to come to a health care provider for help with managing pain. However, because of their frequent ED visits and their need for opioids to treat their severe pain, they may be considered "drug seeking" or "frequent flyers" by some practitioners rather than the "relief seekers" they are in actuality.

In an Institute of Medicine (IOM, 2006) article related to ED practice, health care providers who were asked to indicate their beliefs about patients with sickle-cell disease determined that "fear that the patient is a drug abuser," "disbelief in the patient's report of pain," and "fear of opioid prescribing" were among the top respondent choices. In a similar nursing study, 63% of the respondents indicated that they felt drug addiction was developed in the treatment of sickle-cell pain episodes and 30% were hesitant to administer high-dose opioids (Pack-Masbien, Labbe, & Herbet, 2001). Patients with sickle-cell crisis can wait anywhere from 90 minutes to 10 hours for the first doses of analgesic, despite severe-level pain (Tanabe, Myers, & Zosel, 2007).

These attitudes directly affect the treatment that patients with sickle-cell disease receive. In a survey about addiction in the physician groups who care for these patients, 53% of ED physicians and 23% of hematologists believed that 20% of patients with sickle-cell disease are addicted to opiods (Shapiro, Benjamin, & Payne, 1997). If these are the health care providers that most often see these patients, concern about these attitudes needs to be addressed, and education about the pain management of the disease should be used to change attitudes that are counterproductive to adequate pain relief.

Medications

Because of the severity of the pain, the medications most commonly used to treat patients with sickle-cell crisis are opioids in some form. There is some indication that opioid use can contribute to the development of chest syndrome (Buchanan et al., 2005), a condition that can look like a pneumonia. Morphine and hydromorphone are commonly selected because there is an established track record with these medications. Meperidine is not recommended for treating these patients because when the daily dose is limited to 600 mg per day, patients may have renal impairment, and when large doses are required, patients may have the potential for central nervous system (CNS) buildup of normeperidine, a substance that can cause seizures. Additionally, hydration and blood transfusion are used.

Current recommendations include the use of multimodal analgesia with the use of opioids, NSAIDs, and adjuvants (coanalgesics [Ballas, 2007]). The APS (1999) Sickle-Cell Pain Guideline recommends the following:

- Use aggressive pain management to ease pain and help the patient maintain functionality.

- Tailor analgesic regimens to individual patients.
- NSAIDs or acetaminophen can be used for mild to moderate pain or as pain supplemented with an opioid increases.
- Equianalgesic doses of opioids should be prescribed for home use if needed.
- Tapering of opioids is needed to avoid withdrawal syndrome in patients who have been on opioid therapy for longer than 10 days.
- In addition to the medication recommendations, the use of cognitive behavioral therapies to enhance coping and patient education is highly encouraged (APS, 1999).

Other approaches to disease modification and pain management have been trialed. Yaster et al. (1994) used a continuous epidural catheter with a solution of local anesthetic only or in combination with fentanyl to reduce the pain of sickle-cell crisis in nine children. Patient-controlled analgesia is commonly used for patients in crisis who are hospitalized (Gevirtz, 2008). The use of oxygen can be very effective for patients who are experiencing chest syndrome. Steroids have also been used to reduce the inflammatory component of pain generation (Brookoff, 2009).

Disease-modifying treatment includes the use of transfusions, but long-term transfusions are associated with iron overload, which can require chelating treatment (Ballas, 2007). According to an NIH consensus statement, there is strong evidence to support the use of hydroxyurea, an antimetabolite drug, in adult patients with sickle-cell disease, which can decrease severe painful episodes, hospitalizations, number of blood transfusions, and acute chest syndrome (Brawley et al., 2008).

Developing a Comprehensive Plan of Care for the Patient

Developing a plan of care for the patient with sickle-cell disease involves the use of medications, continued reconditioning, and dietary education. For younger patients, the family will need to know about the illness and the triggers of crises. Consultation with dietary and nutritional counselors can help the young patient understand the need for adequate nutrition and continued hydration. Although the physical toll is great, the emotional components are also important. Coping with a cyclic illness, depression, and anxiety will all need to be assessed and action must be taken when these conditions occur.

The patient with sickle-cell disease will be a frequent consumer of health care and will have several hospitalizations per year for treating severe-level pain. Some facilities have fast-track protocols that can ease the patients through the system, and other institutions have experimented with the use of day hospital facilities where patients can be seen for an extended period, be stabilized, and then return home.

Educating the Patient

Most patients with sickle-cell disease are young and do not like to seem different than their peers. Their self-image is affected in some of the same ways that children with juvenile diabetes or arthritis see themselves. They know they are different but want to be seen as just one of the group when they are with their peers. Because this is a chronic illness, coping with the condition is merited, although cure is not an achievable goal.

Teaching children with sickle-cell disease about what triggers a crisis can help them learn to detect signs and symptoms early in the crisis period. Teaching the patients about the need for hydration and the effect of weather and temperature changes will help alert patients to any increased pain, fatigue, or weakness that could be signs of an impending crisis.

Adding interventions such as biofeedback, relaxation, imagery, and distraction can be helpful for the patient with sickle-cell disease to cope with both the crisis periods and long-term illness. The patient should be encouraged to participate in exercise that does not stress the physical system but maintains conditioning. If the patient becomes depressed, becomes overly anxious, or has unrelieved fears, a psychological evaluation for counseling may be needed.

Sickle-cell disease is a chronic condition with acute exacerbations or crises. Teaching patients how to cope with the unknown aspects of the illness can help reduce pain and decrease stress and anxiety.

Case Study

Cindy is a 24-year-old patient who has been diagnosed with sickle-cell disease. She knows she had it as a child and remembers being hospitalized for pain management and transfusions. She has a brother who also has the disease, but none of her other four siblings have it. She has been admitted four times during the past year for uncontrolled pain. When she is admitted, she complains of pain in her back, chest, and lower extremities. On this admission, she had chest syndrome and needed to use oxygen intermittently. She rates her pain at 8–10/10 when she needs to move.

When she speaks to you about her pain, she says, "I hate this pain. It has been with me it seems all my life. I get really hopeful when I leave the hospital, always thinking it may be the last time I need to go there for pain treatment. When I am out of the hospital, I rarely hurt. If I do, I can use a little Motrin to get by. When I need to go to the hospital, I need IV drugs and I get sleepy, constipated, and I have to taper down from them for weeks after I leave the hospital. I work and I am afraid to tell them what is wrong with me and that I need opioids to treat my pain. I don't want them to think I am a drug addict. I am not sure of what my future will be at this point." How can you help Cindy deal with her pain management?

Questions to Consider

1. If Cindy continues to need opioids to treat her recurrent pain, does this mean she is addicted to them?
2. What triggers can you educate Cindy about and help to incorporate the material into a plan that can decrease Cindy's crises?

REFERENCES

American Pain Society. (1999). *Guideline for the management of acute and chronic pain in sickle cell disease.* Glenview, IL: Author.

Anie, K. A., & Green, J. (2009). Psychological therapies for sickle cell disease and pain. *Cochrane Database of Systematic Reviews*, 4, accession number 00075320-100000000-01325.

Ballas, S. (2007). Current issues in sickle cell pain and its management. *Hematology*, 97–105.

Ballas, S. (2010). Pain and sickle cell disease. In S. M. Fishman, J. C. Ballantyne, & J. P. Rathmell (Eds.), *Bonica's management of pain*. Philadelphia, PA: Lippincott Williams & Wilkins.

Brawley, O. W., Cornelius, E., Gamble, V. N., Green, B., Inturrisi, C., James, A., . . . Schori, M. (2008). *National Institutes of Health consensus development conference statement: Hydroxyurea treatment for sickle cell disease.* Retrieved from www.guideline.gov

Brookoff, D. (2009). Sickle cell anemia. In H. S. Smith (Ed.), *Current therapy in pain* (pp. 348–353). Philadelphia, PA: Elsevier.

Buchanan, I. D., Woodward, M., & Reed, G. (2005). Opioid selection during sickle cell pain crisis and its impact on the development of acute chest syndrome. *Pediatric Blood Cancer, 45*(5), 716–724.

Elliot, J., & Simpson, M. (2010). Persistent pain management. In *Core curriculum for pain management nursing.* Indianapolis, IN: Kendall Hunt.

Gevirtz, C. (2008). Pain management in patients with sickle cell disease. *Topics in Pain Management, 23*(6), 1–12.

Institute of Medicine. (2006). *The future of emergency care in the United States health system*. Washington, DC: National Academies Press.

Pack-Masbien, A., Labbe, E., & Herbert, D. (2001). Nurses' attitudes and practices in sickle cell disease pain management. *Applied Nursing Research, 14,* 187–192.

Platt, A., Beasley, J., Miller, G., & Eckman, J. (2002). Managing sickle cell pain . . . and all that goes with it. *Nursing 2002, 32*(12), 32HN1–32HN7.

Shapiro, B., Benjamin, L., & Payne, R. (1997). Sickle cell-related pain: Perceptions of medical practitioners. *Journal of Pain & Symptom Management, 15,* 168–174.

Tanabe, P., Myers, R., & Zosel, A. (2007). Emergency department management of acute pain episodes in sickle cell disease. *Academic Emergency Medicine, 14,* 419–425.

Yaster, M., Tobin, J. R., Billett, C., Casella, J. F., & Dover, G. (1994). Epidural analgesia in the management of severe vaso-occlusive sickle cell crisis. *Pediatrics, 93*(2), 310–315.

ADDITIONAL RESOURCES

Lazio, M., Costells, H., Courtney, M., Martinovitch, Z., Myers, R., Zosel, A., & Tanabe, P. (2010). A comparison of analgesic management for emergency department patients with sickle cell disease and renal colic. *Clinical Journal of Pain, 26*(3), 199–205.

Oesina, V., Bellini, S., Delaney, C., Bacarro, N., Lundquist, K., D'Angelo, S., & Goodrich, S. (2010). Evidence-based sickle cell pain management in the emergency department. *Advanced Emergency Nursing Journal, 32*(2), 102–111.

Payne, R. (2008). Sickle cell anemia and pain: Will data prevail over beliefs? *Annals of Emergency Medicine, 53*(5), 596–597.

17

Patients With Active Substance Abuse or a History of Substance Abuse

THE PROBLEM OF SUBSTANCE ABUSE

Consider the position of the health care provider who has an established patient–provider relationship with a patient who has a complicated medical history. One of the biggest problems with the patient is difficulty in managing pain. You may have used the best opioid or the dose may be too low on first consideration so dose increases have been made but nothing you do seems to make the pain better. The patient's genetic makeup for medication metabolism may be coming into the picture; however, he or she may also have an unreported history of substance abuse that can affect pain. For these patients, there is a heightened sensitivity to pain and a diminished response to opioid analgesics.

Unless the patient tells you that he or she has a history of substance abuse or is actively using illicit substances, you may find yourself caring for a patient who has difficulty with pain control for no detectable reason. These patients can have a simple procedure, yet complain of severe-level pain that is not controlled with the usual analgesic medications. Even increasing doses of medication for these patients does not seem to improve the level of pain relief, and side effects such as nausea or sedation may start to occur. Although there can be other causes of unrelieved pain, when a patient has a history of substance abuse or is abusing opioids, it tends to remain a problem that reappears when it is least suspected.

The patient who is an addict or has a history of addictive disease may be anyone. He or she can be a trauma patient who is admitted to the hospital or a homemaker housewife who became addicted to pain medication after a past surgery. You cannot tell by looking at the patient whether he or she has a history of addictive disease or if he or she is addicted to an illicit substance. Not all patients are young or show behaviors that indicate addiction. He or she may be an older patient who made a serious mistake with drugs in his or her past who now is still feeling the effects of his or her poor judgment in later life.

Prevalence

Addiction is on the rise. It not only includes the use of "street drugs" such as heroin but also includes the misuse of prescription medications, and teenage abuse of these substances is increasing. The latest government estimate is that prescription drug abuse has increased by 400%. It has become accepted among peer groups and has increased, despite public information announcements that highlight the risks of the practice.

The term *psychotherapeutics* is used as a general term to indicate the categories of drugs that include pain relievers, tranquilizers, stimulants, and sedatives (ASPMN, 2010). The most popular drugs abused by teenagers and young adults are the following:

- hydrocodone (Vicodin)—about 1 in 5 young people
- oxycodone (Oxycontin)—10%
- Drugs for attention deficit disorder, such as methylphenidate (Ritalin) or amphetamine and dextroamphetamine (Adderall)—10% (Generation Rx—Partnership for a Drug-Free America)

Where are these young people obtaining their drugs? Most commonly from a medicine chest at home or in a friend's house; from a relative or friend; from a doctor, a drug dealer, or a stranger; or via the Internet (SAMHSA, 2006). By 2004, the average American teenager had abused a prescription pain reliever in greater numbers than those who used ecstasy, cocaine, crack, or LSD (Generation Rx).

Addiction is not only for the young members of our society. It can be found in patients of any age. In the period from 1992 to 2003, prescription drug abuse in the general population increased from 7.8 million to 15.1 million and rose at a rate that is seven times faster than the increase in the United States population (Under the Counter, 2005).

It is unfortunate, but health care providers will undoubtedly find they have undetected addicts within their patient groups and more with a history of addiction.

Terms

Dealing with patients who have addiction or a history of addiction requires an understanding of the terms *addiction*, *dependency*, *tolerance*, and *pseudoaddiction*.

Addiction is characterized by the four Cs:

- Continued use despite harm
- Impaired control over the drug
- Craving
- Compulsive use (AAAPM, APS, ASAM, 2001; Savage, Covington, Heit, Hunt, Joranson, & Scholl, 2001).

The formal definition of addiction is a primary chronic and neurobiologic disease influenced by genetic, psychosocial, and environmental factors (Savage et al., 2001). Drug addicts are driven to look for and find the substance that they favor. They are not concerned with the effect that the drug is having on their lives; they just know that they need it and will go to any lengths to find and use it. To the drug addicts, the pleasure stimulus that they get from using their drug is worth all that they sacrifice.

Dependency, on the other hand, is a natural phenomenon that occurs with regular use of a medication. All patients who take opioids for more than 30 days become dependent. It is a state of adaptation manifested by a drug class–specific withdrawal syndrome that can be caused by abrupt cessation, rapid dose reductions, or a decrease in the blood level of the drug by the administration of an antagonist (Savage et al., 2001). The patients who are dependent on opioids for pain relief are *not* addicted. They are simply using the medication to continue with their normal activities of living, working, or pursuing a career. It is not correct to label dependent patients as addicted or drug seeking.

Clinical Pearl

The rate of addiction for primary care patients who are using long-term opioid therapy to control their pain is estimated to be 5%. *All* addicts are dependent on their opioid substance of abuse, but not all dependent patients are addicts.

When making chart notes on opioid-dependent patients, do not label them as addicts, and indicate that they are working toward the goal of treatment using the opioids as a part of their treatment plan.

Tolerance is a state of adaptation in which an effect of the medication, such as pain relief, diminishes over time. These patients typically have good pain relief for a period but then start to complain of increased pain. The new pain may be the result of increased activity related to their pain control or just an adaptation mechanism that the patient has no control over. Tolerance does not indicate addiction. It simply means that one or more of the medication effects, such as nausea, sedation, and pain relief, have decreased. Increasing doses may reduce the pain level, or an opioid rotation, as described in the medication section, may be needed to restore adequate pain relief.

Pseudoaddiction is the development of patient behaviors that mimic what health care providers perceive as drug seeking, such as clock watching and frequent requests for specific pain medications. In reality, this behavior is a result of undertreated pain. Once the pain is treated adequately, the drug related behaviors disappear.

The Difference Between Addictive and Aberrant Drug-Taking Behaviors

Patients who are using long-term opioid analgesics can exhibit behaviors that appear to be a developing addiction but, in truth, are classed as aberrant, not addictive. These behaviors are motivated by various conditions, such as past experiences with the health care system or undertreated pain. Some behaviors that are considered aberrant but not addictive include the following:

- Requesting specific drugs
- Aggressive complaining about the need for higher doses
- Drug hoarding during periods of reduced symptoms
- Unapproved use of the drug to treat another symptom
- Reporting psychic effects not intended by the provider
- Unsanctioned dose escalation once or twice
- Obtaining similar drugs from other medical sources
- Resistance to change in therapy associated with tolerable adverse effects, with expressions of anxiety about the return of severe symptoms (Fine & Portnoy, 2007)

When patients exhibit behaviors that are more predictive of addiction, it is a very different situation. The behaviors are more pronounced and severe in nature. They indicate the lack of control that the patient has with drugs, and often these behaviors manifest very quickly if the health care provider recognizes danger signs and starts to control opioid use. Behaviors that can indicate a developing addiction include the following:

- Injecting or snorting oral formulations for quicker onset
- Forging prescriptions
- Selling or stealing prescription drugs
- Obtaining prescription drugs from nonmedical sources, such as drug dealers, other addicts, or over the Internet

- Concurrent use of illicit drugs with the prescribed opioids
- Unsanctioned and continued dose escalations
- Recurrent and frequent prescription losses
- Deterioration in personal life and appearing more unkempt or appearing intoxicated
- Solid resistance to changes in opioid therapy, despite demonstrated harm (Fine & Portnoy, 2007)

Once these addictive behaviors start, the health care provider must investigate the source and begin more aggressive urine screening, prescription control, pill counts, and mandating compliance with the opioid treatment agreement described in the following sections. Tools for estimating risk with opioid use are also described in the following section. These tools can help the health care provider determine which patients may experience difficulty with opioids and start more stringent monitoring earlier in the treatment period.

Assessing and Screening

When performing a physical examination on an addicted patient, look for signs of current drug use, track marks on the arms, needle marks from injection between toes or in tattoos that can hide the injection marks, or skin-popping scars from subcutaneous injection of substances such as heroin. Inspect the nares for signs of excoriation or irritation from snorted drugs such as cocaine. Patients who are smoking marijuana or heroin may come in frequently with complaints of cough or shortness of breath. With prolonged heroin abuse using highly contaminated drugs, the patients may have a chest X-ray with heavy scarring, indicating a "heroin lung," in which lung tissues have become blocked with the contaminants. Once obvious signs of drug abuse are identified, a more complete physical workup, including HIV testing and hepatitis tests, is indicated.

Patients who have had extended exposure to opioids or used illicit substances such as heroin will have a decreased response to opioid medications. They will also have increased sensitivity to pain.

Given these characteristics, assessing pain will be difficult. Patients with an addiction history will need more medication but may continue to consistently report high levels of pain.

When discussing the pain complaint, recognize that addicted patients have often been misidentified, overlabeled, and undertreated. They are less open to discussion about pain management, fearing they will again be labeled as addicted and possibly denied treatment with opioids. Dependent patients have had similar experiences in which they have been labeled as addicts when, in reality, they are dependent on opioid medication to relieve their daily pain. Some health care providers see the development of tolerance as a sure sign that the patient is becoming addicted to opioid analgesics. Understanding the difference between the three conditions can help clarify the assessment process.

Using a simple numeric rating scale (NRS), with 0–10 for acute injuries, can be all that is needed for pain assessment and tracking the efficacy of pain management medications and interventions in acute care. Two simple and easy-to-use screens are the *CAGE* and the *TRAUMA*. They work well for patients who are admitted for care after accidents or are being seen in the emergency department for acute pain when alcohol abuse or substance abuse is suspected.

To assess a patient using the *CAGE*, simply ask the patient the following four questions:

- Have you ever tried to CUT down on your alcohol or drug use?
- Have people ANNOYED you by commenting on or criticizing your drinking or drug use?
- Have you ever felt bad or GUILTY about your drinking or drug use?
- Have you ever needed an EYE OPENER first thing in the morning to steady your nerves or get rid of a hangover?

This type of simple screen takes only a few minutes and can give the health care provider an idea about either alcohol or substance abuse. The more positive responses the patient gives, the greater the likelihood that the patient has an alcohol or drug abuse problem (Chou et al., 2009).

To assess a patient using the *TRAUMA* screen, ask the patient the five questions that are related to the patient's injury history. Since age 18, have you:

- Had any fractures or dislocations to your bones or joints, excluding sports injuries?
- Been injured in a traffic accident?
- Injured your head, excluding sports injuries?
- Been in a fight or assaulted while intoxicated?
- Been injured while intoxicated?

If the patient answers "yes" to two or more of the questions, there is a high potential for abuse (Chou et al., 2009).

The *CAGE* and the *TRAUMA* screen give the health care provider an idea of the potential for substance abuse. For more detailed assessment, the Brief Pain Impact Questionnaire (BPIQ) described in Chapter 4 provides an interview technique for covering most questions needed for an initial visit assessment including substance abuse.

More extensive screens for determining risks associated with opioid prescribing have been developed. These tools are most appropriate for long-term prescribing of opioids, but some tools can identify those patients who will have more problems when opioids are used for analgesia.

- The Opioid Risk Tool is used to determine what the risk is when the patient is prescribed opioids for pain. There is a list of simple questions related to family history of substance abuse, personal history of substance abuse, age, history of any preadolescent sexual abuse, any psychological disease, and depression. The patient who scores 0–3 is considered low risk, 4–7 is considered moderate risk, and a patient scoring greater than 8 in this screen is considered most likely to develop aberrant behaviors with opioid use. This tool is designed for determining opioid risk prior to starting opioid therapy (D'Arcy, 2010a; Passik, Kirsh, & Casper, 2008).
- The Screener and Opioid Assessment for Patients with Pain-Revised (SOAPP-R) is a tool designed to screen patients who are being considered for long-term opioid therapy. It consists of 14 questions related to substance abuse history, medication-related behaviors, antisocial behaviors, doctor–patient relationships, and personal care

and lifestyle issues. A score of 8 or greater indicates a high risk of abuse or misuse (D'Arcy, 2010a; Passik et al., 2008).

- Diagnosis, Intractability, Risk, and Efficacy (DIRE) Score allows a provider to determine if the patient is a good candidate for opioid therapy. It has four categories: diagnosis, intractability, risk, and efficacy. A score of 14 or higher indicates that the patient is a good candidate for opioid therapy. Patients with lower scores are not good candidates for opioid therapy (Passik et al., 2008).
- Current Opioid Misuse Measure (COMM) is a 17-item self-report tool that is used to identify aberrant behaviors for patients who are currently on opioid therapy. The COMM as a newer tool can identify emotional or psychiatric issues, evidence of lying, appointment patterns, and medication misuse or noncompliance. This tool is designed for use when aberrant behaviors increase in frequency (Butler et al., 2007; D'Arcy, 2010b).

These tools should always be considered only as a part of the assessment process and should be used in conjunction with standard pain assessments and consideration of the total patient history. For patients being seen in clinics as outpatients, the NRS is adequate for assessing and reassessing pain at each visit and tracking the effectiveness of the medications being used. The long-term care of these patients may necessitate more extensive screening and documentation.

The Pain Assessment and Documentation Tool is helpful in tracking patients who are on opioid therapy for pain management. It is a tool that is based on the four As:

- **Analgesia**—pain ratings during the week, a percentage of pain that has been relieved, and whether the amount of pain relief makes a difference in the patient's life
- **Activities of daily living**—assessments of physical functioning, relationships, moods, sleep, and overall functioning
- **Adverse events**—side effects such as nausea, fatigue, itching, constipation, drowsiness, or mental clouding
- **Aberrant drug-related behavior**—purposeful oversedation, abusing alcohol, or other illicit drugs, requests frequent early renewals, increases dose without authorization, changes routes of administration, and requests prescriptions from other doctors

This tool can indicate that the opioid therapy is producing positive results for the patient or is not providing the expected outcomes. Tracking the patient over time in a consistent format can highlight early indications of change as it occurs, allowing the health care provider to adjust the current medication regimen or taper the patients off the current medications.

Developing a Plan of Care

Before developing a comprehensive treatment plan for the patient, there are some items to consider.

- Do I have enough information to diagnose and formulate a comprehensive plan of care?
- Is a trial of opioids merited, and, if so, what are the risks and benefits?
- Can I treat this patient alone?
- Do I need additional consultants? Who would they be?
- Do I need help to manage the patient?
- Does the patient require care that exceeds my resources? (Smith, Fine, & Passik, 2009)

In most cases, the patient who is an addict or has a history of substance abuse will need a team approach. For trauma patients admitted to acute care, consultation with a pain team or pain specialist is helpful. In primary care, practitioners skilled in dealing with addiction, psychologists, pain specialists, social workers, psychiatrists, and rehabilitation specialists can all be considered as part of the team. Careful planning and teams of specialists can help to ensure that the plan of care includes all that is needed and that it will provide the most benefit with the least amount of risk.

Drug addicts and patients with a history of substance abuse will need higher doses of medication to control their pain. This is a result of the physiologic changes that take place with substance abuse or long-term opioid use. They also have a heightened sensitivity to pain and a decreased response to opioid medications. Because of these changes, opioid doses will need to be higher than the current doses of opioids for chronic pain, and for the addicted patient, an estimation of medication will have to be made from the patient's report of substance used on a daily basis.

These questions can be difficult to ask, but they will need to be discussed to determine what amount of medication will be needed to treat pain and avoid withdrawal syndrome. To develop a plan of care for these patients requires a time commitment to deal not only with the clinical issues but also with the psychological coping and addictive personality. As outpatients, these patients require close monitoring, frequent urine screens, and careful prescription management. In the acute care setting, the focus should be on treating the patient's pain and making appropriate referrals for outpatient services when the patient is discharged. Some patients with a history of substance abuse will be very resistant to using opioids, fearing readdiction. For these patients, a combination of therapies, including regional techniques (see Chapter 14), nonopioid medications, and careful opioid use, can provide adequate pain control.

The treatment plans for patients with addictive disease are very comprehensive. They should be individualized and spell out the risk and benefits clearly to both the patients and the health care providers involved in the patient's care. An integral part of the treatment plan for outpatients is a treatment agreement that spells out the terms of opioid use. These agreements are essential for protecting the prescriber from any misunderstandings or legal issue, and they provide the patients with the information they need when opioids are being used to treat pain. These agreements define addiction, dependency, and tolerance. They detail what medications are being prescribed, how they should be used, and who should prescribe them. The agreements also detail what the penalty will be if illicit drugs are detected in random drug screens and what the options are for the prescriber should this occur. Samples of treatment agreements are available at http://www.painmed.org

Random drug screens or urine drug monitoring (UDM) is an essential part of the treatment agreement and it should be random, not scheduled. Starting with a baseline urine screen when opioids are started can be helpful in establishing the procedure for UDM. The response of the health care provider to finding illicit substances not prescribed for the patient in the urine screen should be clearly defined in the treatment agreement.

Urine drug screens can detect and identify the presence of a substance or a metabolite that indicates that a particular drug is present. Some medications clear the urine quickly, whereas others, such as phenobarbital, may be present for longer periods. The use of urine screens is effective for determining the presence of a particular drug, but it can also provide a false-positive or false-negative result. Medications such as antibiotics can cause a false-positive result. There is usually a 1–3 day period when drugs are present in the urine and can be detected. Some drugs, such as methamphetamine, benzodiazepines, fentanyl, heroin, and most opiates, clear the urine within 1–5 days, whereas other drugs, such as methadone, phenobarbital, phencyclidine, and propoxyphene, are present for longer periods, around 7–14 days.

Using a urine screen for maintaining an opioid agreement can indicate that the appropriate drug is being used and no illicit drugs are being used. It can also prove that the prescribed drug is not present in the urine, which may indicate diversion. If there is any concern with the results of a urine screen, a gas chromatography test can further define the findings of the urine screen and give more specific information. Treating a patient with a history of addiction or with active substance abuse can be very challenging. Adding in a significant complaint of pain heavily complicates the patient's needs. It is important when treating this type of patient to use the documentation process to indicate why the opioids are being prescribed and what the benefits have been. In this way both the patient and prescriber's best interests are preserved.

Case Study

Sabrina K., 18 years old, is admitted through the emergency department. She was a passenger in a car that was hit from the side at high speed. She is unconscious, so no medical history can be obtained from her. She has multiple fractures on her lower extremities, a compression fracture in her lumbar vertebra, and a closed head injury. She was an unbelted passenger and has sustained a significant concussion, which will make it difficult to obtain an idea of what happened to her in the accident. When her parents arrive, you ask them about Sabrina's health history. They tell you, "Sabrina has been a model child. She gets all As and Bs at school. She is on the cheerleading squad and plays volleyball in the spring. She has always been such a good child. I don't know how this could have happened to her." You proceed to asking them about her history of substance abuse, and the parents respond, "Why? Sabrina has never used drugs and we have never known her to use alcohol either. Of course, we let her have a little beer or wine at home for special occasions."

When you get Sabrina's urine screen back, she has an elevated alcohol level and is positive for opioids and amphetamines. How will you proceed with Sabrina's care?

Questions to Consider

1. Sabrina is 18. Will you tell her parents about the laboratory results?
2. Once Sabrina is stable and able to discuss her drug use, how will you proceed with opening up the discussion?
3. What issues will you face in treating Sabrina's pain?
4. After two weeks the nurses tell you Sabrina won't go to physical therapy because she hurts too much. You are using a long-acting opioid with short-acting opioid for breakthrough pain. Will increasing her dose be beneficial? What other options should you consider?

REFERENCES

American Academy of Pain Medicine, American Pain Society, & American Society of Addiction Medicine. (2001). Definitions related to the use of opioids for the treatment of pain. *Wisconsin Medical Journal, 100*(5), 28–29.

American Pain Society. (2008). *Principles of analgesic use in the treatment of acute pain and cancer pain.* Glenview, IL: Author.

American Society of Pain Management Nurses. (2010). Coexisting addiction and pain. In B. St. Marie (Ed.), *Core curriculum for pain management nursing.* Indianapolis, IN: Kendall Hunt.

Butler, S. F., Budman, S. H., Fernandez, K. C., Houle, B., Benoit, C., Katz, N., & Jamison, R. N. (2007). Development and validation of the Current Opioid Misuse Measure. *Pain, 130*(1–2), 144–156.

Chou, R., Fanciullo, G. J., Fine, P. G., Adler, J., Ballantyne, J., Davies, P., . . . Donovan, M. I. (2009). Clinical guidelines for the use of opioid therapy in chronic no cancer pain. *Pain, 10*(2), 113–130.

D'Arcy, Y. (2010a). *Pain assessment in core curriculum for pain management nursing.* Indianapolis, IN: Kendall Hunt.

D'Arcy, Y. (2010b). Treating pain in addicted patient: Great challenge, greater reward. *Advance for Nurse Practitioners, 18*(5), 20–25.

Generation Rx—Partnership for a Drug-Free America. Retrieved from http://pharmacy.osu.edu/outreach/generation-rx

The National Center on Addiction and Substance Abuse at Columbia University. (2005). *Under the counter: The diversion and abuse of controlled prescription drugs in the U.S.* Retrieved from www.casacolumbia.org

Passik, S., Kirsh, K. L., & Casper, D. (2008). Addiction-related assessment tools and pain management: Instruments for screening, treatment planning, and monitoring compliance. *Pain Medicine, 9*(S2), S145–S166.

Savage, S., Covington, E., Heit, H., Hunt, J., Joranson, D., & Scholl, S. (2001). *Definitions related to the use of opioids for the treatment of pain: A consensus document from the American Academy of Pain Medicine, the American Pain Society, and the American Society of Addiction Medicine.* Glenview, IL: American Association of Physicists in Medicine.

Smith, H., Fine, P., & Passik, S. (2009). *Opioid risk management tools and tips.* New York: Oxford University Press.

Substance Abuse and Mental Health Services Administration. (2006). *Results from the 2005 National Survey on Drug Use and Health: National findings* (Office of Applied Studies, NSDUH Series H-30. DHHS Publication No. SMA 06-4194. Rockville, MD). Retrieved from http://oas.samhsa.gov/nsduhLatest.htm

Webster, L., & Dove, L. (2007). *Avoiding opioid abuse while managing pain.* North Branch, MN: Sunrise River Press.

ADDITIONAL RESOURCE

Passik, S., & Kirsh, K. (2009). Pain in the substance abuse population. In H. S. Smith (Ed.), *Current therapy in pain.* Philadelphia, PA: Elsevier.

18

Abdominal Pain

PREVALENCE OF ABDOMINAL PAIN

Abdominal pain is a common occurrence in most acute care settings. It can be the result of flu, constipation, or more serious conditions, such as small bowel obstruction, perforated viscous, or an exacerbation of Crohn's disease. No matter what the cause, the diagnosis and treatment options for pain can be limited. If the patient is made nothing by mouth (NPO), the treatment options shrink even further.

In the past, pain medications were often withheld from patients who complained of abdominal pain in fear that giving opioids might mask symptoms that could be useful for diagnosis (Manterola et al., 2008). Newer information indicates that providing pain medication to a patient with abdominal pain can lead to not only reduced pain for the patient but also greater accuracy with diagnosis (Manterola et al., 2008).

Abdominal pain is considered to be one of the top three diagnoses for patients who are seen in emergency departments (EDs) and accounts for 7.5 million ED visits annually (U.S. Centers for Disease Control and Prevention, 2004). For 35% to 51% of these patients, no specific etiology is found to explain the cause of the pain. However, up to one third of the patients with abdominal pain require surgical intervention (Irvin, 1989; Klinkman, 1996).

Abdominal pain has both somatic and visceral elements. It can also be referred from a site that is distant from the source of the pain.

- *Visceral pain* is sensed as a diffuse type of pain that does not localize and covers a large area of the abdomen. It can be the result of ischemia, inflammation, distension of the hollow viscous, or capsular distension of solid viscera (Rosati & Stain, 2009).
- *Somatic pain* is sensed as a sharp type of pain that is lateralized (Rosati & Stain, 2009). It localizes to a specific area of the abdomen (Mayer & Wong, 2010). Somatic pain arises from a different sensory locale, the peritoneum.
- *Referred pain* originates in a site that is different from the perceived source of the pain. A common type of referred pain is subscapular pain caused by gallbladder disease or back pain resulting from the pancreas (Rosati & Stain, 2009).

Knowing what type of pain the patient is experiencing can help determine the source of the pain. When assessing patients for abdominal pain, it is important to obtain a full assessment that includes location, radiation, quality, associated symptoms, onset, and duration. Conducting a complete history that includes any significant comorbidities, recent travel, and previous illnesses and medications is needed. The physical examination includes inspecting the abdomen, palpating all four quadrants with deep palpation, percussion, and auscultation. Tinkling bowel sounds may indicate a small bowel obstruction. Rebound tenderness may indicate appendicitis.

DIFFERENTIAL DIAGNOSIS

The options for differential diagnosis with abdominal pain are extensive. Options include a wide range of conditions that can be the source of the pain, including the following:

- *Generalized pain*—perforated viscus, intestinal obstruction, intestinal ischemia, colitis, pancreatitis, early appendicitis, constipation, ruptured abdominal aortic aneurysm, gastroenteritis, diabetic ketoacidosis, sickle-cell crisis, uremia, leukemia, porphyria, and Munchausen's syndrome

- *Cardiac sources*—aortic dissection, myocardial infarction, aortic aneurysm, pericarditis, myocardial ischemia/infarction, and thoracoabdominal aneurysm/dissection
- *Gastroinstestinal/Endocrine sources*—peptic ulcer, splenic injury, splenic infarction, subphrenic abscess, intestinal obstruction, intestinal ischemia, colitis, pancreatitis, pancreatic pseudocyst, diverticular disease, benign and malignant colonic obstruction, ischemic colitis, subphrenic abscess, liver abscess, hepatobiliary and pancreatic neoplasms, biliary colic, cholesystitis, cholangitis, Fitz-Hugh-Curtis syndrome, appendicitis, inflammatory bowel disease, and gastroenteritis
- *Gastric ulcer sources*—pyelonephritis, renal colic, renal neoplasm, pelvic inflammatory disease, benign and adnexal masses, ectopic pregnancy, and endometriosis
- *Pulmonary sources*—pulmonary embolism and left lower lobe pneumonia
- *Musculoskeletal sources*—abdominal wall hernia, inguinal hernia, herpes zoster, and psoas abscess (Rosati & Stain, 2009)

This comprehensive list contains the main types of differential diagnosis that can be made for abdominal pain. Combining the patient's report of pain with the physical exam and laboratory test can help lead the health care provider to the source of the abdominal pain. In some instances, the pain cannot be diagnosed and only after surgery can the source of the pain be more readily identified.

The use of computed tomography (CT) can improve diagnostic accuracy by 40% to 50% (Esses et al., 2004). Other laboratory tests, such as complete blood count (CBC), electrolytes, urinalysis, and electrocardiogram, are used to rule out infection and organ dysfunction. Although finding the source of the pain is useful for diagnosis, treating the pain is necessary, no matter what the source of the pain.

TREATMENT OPTIONS

Treatment for severe-level abdominal pain will necessitate the use of opioid medications, most commonly given as intravenous (IV) injections. Because opioids can slow bowel function and create an ileus, using a coanalgesic such as IV ketorolac (Toradol), when bleeding is not a contraindication, can help decrease opioid consumption, and improve pain relief. Oral pain medications as described in the medication chart can be used for ambulatory care patients who need short-term pain relief. Always prescribe a laxative for patients who will be taking opioids for pain control, so that constipation does not become a problem. Using complementary techniques for pain relief when the pain is under reasonable control can help the patient to relax.

For postoperative pain relief, a local anesthetic catheter along the incision line can help decrease the pain and assist with movement. Because most abdominal surgery patients require opioids for several days after surgery, either patient-controlled analgesia (PCA) or epidural can be used for pain relief. In a systematic review of nine studies with patients who had intra-abdominal surgery, continuous epidural analgesia was superior for pain relief when compared with PCA, but pruritus was more common (Werawatganon & Charuluxanun, 2009). In another systematic review of epidural analgesia and intravenous opioids after abdominal aortic surgery, epidural was found to provide superior pain relief, and postoperative ventilation times were reduced (Nishimori, Ballantyne, & Low, 2009).

Some patients are admitted for intractable abdominal pain before the source of the pain can be determined. For these patients, using a PCA can help determine how much medication will be needed to control the pain once the patient is able to take oral pain medications. For less severe abdominal pain, the use of IV Toradol is effective for patients who are being seen in the ED, and it can be added to a PCA regimen for opioid-sparing effect. Mild analgesics, such as those on the first level of the analgesic ladder, can also be used. The use of antispasmodic agents has only low-level support for use in such conditions as irritable bowel syndrome (IBS; Mayer & Wong, 2010).

DEVELOPING A PLAN OF CARE

The plan of care for patients with abdominal pain should be multimodal and include not only analgesics but also the use of complementary techniques and psychological assessment to identify stress, episode triggers, and comorbidities such as abuse.

- Obtain a full history from the patients that includes any recent travel or any similar complaints that have happened in the past.
- Obtain stool cultures if diarrhea is one of the symptoms.
- Perform a complete blood panel for electrolytes, hematology, and hepatitis.
- Perform a full physical examination that includes palpation and auscultation and note any rebound tenderness or usual swelling.
- Ask the patient to rate his or her pain and provide a suitable medication for pain.
- If more extensive testing is required, order a CT to determine if there are any masses, nodes, or infectious process.
- Once the diagnosis is made, discuss treatment options with the patient and provide patient education about the specific condition.

PATIENT EDUCATION

Patients who have abdominal pain will need education on diet, medication use, and training in techniques to reduce stress. Patient education should include the following points:

- *Special diets*—Some patients with abdominal pain will need special diets, such as low-fiber diets. Patients should be referred to a dietician, who can help provide information and recipes that patients can use.
- *Constipation and bowel regimens*—Patients should be taught about adequate bowel regimens. Recurrent constipation can be painful and difficult to manage. Teaching the patients about the different types of laxatives will help provide success with the recommended laxative regimen.
- *Comorbid conditions*—Patients with a condition such as Crohn's disease have a chronic condition that can reoccur. Informing the patients about resources that they can access for support can help the patients cope with the chronic illness. Providing information on disease-specific diets is especially important for patients with this condition.

- *Conveying reasonable pain control expectations*—Creating the correct expectation for medications with a patient who has recurrent abdominal pain can be one of the most important aspects of care. If patients feel that opioids are all that works for them, they will expect increases in doses and continued opioids to manage their pain. Teaching patients about the impact of chronic opioid use that requires increasing dosages, which may not be in the patient's best interest, can go far in making hospitalizations less traumatic.
- *Surgical patients*—These patients should be given opioids to facilitate activity such as walking, which can restore bowel function sooner after surgery. If opioids are being provided for pain control, the expectation that it will facilitate patient activity early in the postoperative period should be explained to the patient early in the hospitalization.

Treating patients with abdominal pain can be very frustrating because there are so many options for the source of the pain. Listening to the patient's report of the pain and reviewing the history can be the best way to help diagnose the pain. Patients with abdominal pain can be treated with opioids, but careful monitoring for continued use and adverse effects such as ileus is needed. As always, patients who are prescribed opioids should also be placed on a bowel regimen so that constipation can be avoided.

Case Study

Rose J., a 45-year-old patient, is being seen in the ED for a reoccurrence of abdominal pain. She complains of diffuse pain that is at an 8/10 level. It is constant and sharp. She is holding her abdomen and rocking back and forth on the stretcher. She is nauseated and vomits undigested food. Her abdomen is distended and hard. She is tearful and cries intermittently. She tells you, "This time the pain is so much worse. It gets started and won't stop. I don't know what to do to make it better. Nothing I tried worked. It's been this way since last night. I just can't stand it any more." The ED provider does not want to give Rose any pain medication, because he feels it may mask her symptoms. What would you do?

Questions to Consider

1. Is withholding medication the appropriate decision?
2. What types of medication would be best for Rose at this point?
3. You learn that Rose had abdominal surgery last year. You suspect she has abdominal adhesions that have caused a small bowel obstruction. She has had some long-term pain and is being seen now with this intense exacerbation of her pain. How will you treat the pain long term after her surgical treatment?
4. Is there a role for coanalgesic medications in her treatment plan, such as those for neuropathic pain or complementary techniques?

REFERENCES

Esses, D., Birnbaum, A., Bijur, P., Shah, S., Gleyzer, A., & Gallagher, E. J. (2004). Ability of CT to alter decision making in elderly patients with acute abdominal pain. *American Journal of Emergency Medicine, 22*, 270–272.

Irvin, T. T. (1989). Abdominal pain: A surgical audit of 1190 emergency admissions. *British Journal of Surgery, 76*, 1121–1125.

Klinkman, M. S. (1996). Episodes of care for abdominal pain in a primary care practice. *Archives of Family Medicine, 5*, 279–285.

Manterola, C., Astudillo, P., Losada, H., Pineda, V., Sanheunza, A., & Vial, M. (2008). Analgesia in patients with acute abdominal pain. *The Cochrane Collaboration.*

Mayer, E., & Wong, H. (2010). *Bonica's management of pain* (4th ed.). Philadelphia, PA: Lippincott Williams & Wilkins.

Nishimori, M., Ballantyne, J. C., & Low, J. H. (2009). Epidural pain relief versus systemic opioid-based pain relief for abdominal aortic surgery. *Cochrane Database of Systematic Reviews*, 1.

Rosati, C., & Stain, S. (2009). Abdominal pain. In H. S. Smith (Ed.), *Current therapy in pain.* Philadelphia, PA: Elsevier.

U.S. Centers for Disease Control and Prevention. (2004). *National hospital ambulatory care survey 2004 emergency department summary*. Retrieved from http://www.cdc.gov/nchs/data/ad/ad372.pdf

Werawatganon, T., & Charuluxanun, S. (2009). Patient-controlled intravenous opioid analgesia versus continuous epidural analgesia for pain after intra-abdominal surgery. *Cochrane Database of Systematic Reviews*, 1.

19

Emergency Room, Trauma, and Critical Care Patients With Pain

EMERGENCY ROOM PAIN

This chapter provides some basic information on acute pain management for critical care patients in various settings. More complete information on this patient population can be found in *Compact Clinical Guide to Critical Care, Trauma and Emergency Pain Management: An Evidence-Based Approach for Nurses* (forthcoming from Springer Publishing Company).

The patient seeking health care through an emergency room (ER) comes into the hospital for a wide variety of reasons. It may be that something has just occurred that brings the patient in for treatment, such as a fall with injuries or a bleeding cut. Or it may be that the patient has been suffering for a headache for days and the pain has become too much for the patient to endure, so he or she comes into the ER seeking pain relief. Or, the patient may have been in an accident and requires trauma services. One of the fastest growing ER populations are those individuals who lack health insurance and use the ER as their primary care clinic.

The prevalence of pain among ER patients is very high at 78% (Cordell et al., 2002; Todd, 2010). Some of these patients come in for help with acute conditions but 40% have chronic pain and require more extensive medical management. Results of a national survey indicate that there are 24 million adults with chronic pain who make 12 million ER visits as a result of exacerbations of chronic pain conditions (Todd, Cowan, & Kelly, 2010).

Because of the high rates of pain and patients with substance abuse, health care providers who work in the emergency department (ED) are torn between relieving the patient's pain and not contributing to an addictive disease. This is also more pertinent to this area of practice because health care providers in the ED prescribe some of the most commonly diverted opioid medications. Using prescription monitoring programs is one technique that can help these health care providers track opioid data for specific patients and help to determine the true state of the opioid use for the patient. These programs collate opioid-prescribing data from surrounding pharmacies to help determine who has prescribed opioid medications for specific patients in the recent past.

Another issue with treating pain in the ED is the wait that patients with pain experience. Most EDs have a target time that is set to decrease patient wait times. Findings from a national survey indicate that one in four patients waited longer than the target time to be evaluated by the ED health care provider (Horwitz & Bradley, 2009). More emergent patients are triaged and seen quickly, whereas those with more chronic complaints wait longer to be seen.

When the patient is seen by the ED health care provider, asking questions about the pain can be reassuring to the patient and has resulted in high satisfaction ratings by patients. Simply asking about the patient's pain seems to indicate concern (Todd & Miner, 2010). Analgesic regimens in the ED are fairly simple. If the pain is minor, nonopioids such as nonsteroidal anti-inflammatory drugs (NSAIDs) are used. Moderate pain may be treated with mild-to-moderate level opioids because the patient will leave the department once he or she is treated. Severe level pain can be treated with intravenous (IV) medications, followed by a prescription for oral analgesics. The intramuscular route is not recommended for pain medication because absorption rates are not predictable (American Pain Society [APS], 2008). The top 10 medications provided in emergency visits were opioids, NSAIDs, nonnarcotic analgesics, antipyretics, antiemetics, antihistamines, sedatives, cephalosporins, antiasthmatics, and penicillins (Todd & Miner, 2010). Depending on the patient's disposition, appropriate pain medications can be provided to include patient-controlled analgesia (PCA) or epidurals for those patients with severe pain being admitted to the hospital. Providing the right medications can help promote earlier patient recovery and a faster return to his or her normal level of function.

Trauma Pain

Trauma patients arrive at the ER as unknown. The patients were perhaps on their way to work and were in an automobile accident, thus bringing them into an ER. They are not prepared for what has happened to them, they "come as they are" and it is the job of the trauma team to assess and care for their pain and injuries.

One of the most common traumas seen in community hospitals is blunt thoracic trauma (BTT). BTT can be caused by patient falls or automobile accidents where undue pressure to the chest results in broken ribs, soft tissue damage, or injuries to the boney area of the thorax. This type of trauma commonly results in multiple rib fractures or flail chest injuries. These injuries can severely impact respiratory status and may even result in a pneumothorax or hemothorax. Common causes of BTT include crushing from steering wheels and seatbelts in cars; tables and counter edges in homes; and trees, guard rails, or windshields when patients are ejected from vehicles. The resultant injuries can include injuries to the following:

- Spleen and pancreas
- Liver
- Small and large bowel
- Cardiac and pulmonary systems
- Facial structures

To further complicate matters, very often the patient with a BTT will have also sustained a head injury, which makes the assessment process much more difficult. This type of injury can also limit the use of opioids to treat pain in efforts to maintain cerebral oxygenation levels.

The methods that are used to diagnose BTT are computed tomography (CT), diagnostic peritoneal lavage (DPL), and focused abdominal sonography for trauma (FAST) (American College of

Emergency Physicians [ACEP], 2002). In approximately 19% of patients diagnosed with BTT, abdominal tenderness was not present (ACEP, 2002).

The outcomes used to determine the success of treating BTT are ventilator days, length of hospitalization, subjective pain perception, mortality, respiratory depression, and incidence of complication rate (Blunt Thoracic Trauma Guideline, 2004). Treatment option recommendations for treating BTT from the 2004 guidelines to provide the best outcomes are as follows:

Level 1: Use of epidural analgesia provides maximum pain relief; improves subjective pain report; and reduces respiratory depression, constipation, and somnolence.

Level 2: Use of opioid and local anesthetic combinations is for patients who are 65 years and older and younger patients with four or more rib fractures. Outcomes derived with this therapy are decreased ventilator days, decreased intensive care unit (ICU) stay, and overall length of hospitalization.

Level 3: Use of intravenous opioids is in divided doses (if not contraindicated), intercostal blockade, and intrapleural and paravertebral analgesia.

Some patients are the best candidates for these therapies, such as the older adults, patients with comorbid conditions, and especially those with cardiopulmonary disease and diabetes. When these patients are being treated for BTT, a subjective response to pain control is the expected outcome. No matter what the age, providing adequate analgesia for patients with BTT will improve the chances for recovery and decrease the time it takes to return to baseline functional status.

Critical Care Pain Management

Patients who are in critical care can often have their pain management needs overlooked, given the severity of their medical condition. Intravenous opioids have long been used in these patients, but medical conditions such as renal disease or liver dysfunction can limit their use. Because there is a lack of research support for pain management in this patient group, many times the patient's pain management needs are overlooked, especially with the critical nature of the patient's condition.

It is important to remember that the patient comes into the critical care setting bringing all of his or her current pain management issues. All critically ill patients have the right to adequate analgesia and management of their pain (Jacobi et al., 2002). Some of the patients will have low back pain, rheumatoid arthritis, or other chronic painful conditions that are not helped by being confined to a bed. The procedures and care being provided can also be painful, as illustrated in the Thunder II Project (Puntillo et al., 2001), where procedures and turning that had been provided pain scores that were higher than expected.

A large number of patients in the critical care setting will be ventilated, which has been identified as painful by patients. To maintain the ventilation, patients are sedated with a sedative agent, such as propofol (Diprivan) or midazolam (Versed), combined with an opioid, such as morphine or fentanyl (Sublimaze). Because the patient in the intensive care unit (ICU) is under physiological stress, normal organ function is impaired at some level. Using medications on a continuous basis can also impact the way the drug is processed. For example, fentanyl is noted to have a quick onset and quick offset when given as a bolus dose; however, the half-life of the medication when used as a continuous infusion for sedation can stretch to 13 hours (Erstad et al., 2009).

When pain is unrelieved in the critical care unit, there can be consequences that reach beyond the pain itself. Some systemic and physiologic effects include the following:

- Immune system—decreased immune response and ability to fight infection
- Cardiovascular—increased oxygen demand on heart muscle, creating stress and ischemia
- Renal—water and sodium retention
- Endocrine—hyperglycemia and hypotension
- Respiratory—hypoxia, ventilator dysfunction, increased pneumonia risk, and atelectasis
- Psychological—depression, fatigue, and anxiety
- Hematologic—gastrointestinal bleeding and thromboembolic disease (Mularski, Sessler, & Schmidt, 2010).

Given the serious nature of the consequences, providing adequate analgesia for critically ill patients is highly important.

Many procedures experienced by critically ill patients are painful, as indicated in the results of the Thunder II Project. Suctioning, turning in bed, chest tube insertion, and femoral line removal all produce pain. A behavioral pain scale, such as the Payen Behavioral Pain Scale (BPS) or the Critical Care Observation Tool, should be used to assess pain in patients who are unable to self-report. The pain assessment should be followed with the use of an analgesic agent that is meant to control pain at the level of the assessment. Controlling pain in these patients can help to decrease stress and potentially decrease ventilation time.

Just because a critically ill patient is sedated does not mean that his or her pain is controlled. Additionally, sedation does not mean that the patient will not remember the events experienced when under sedation. In a study of critical care patients who were sedated and ventilated, 55% had recall of the events and pain, although they were perceived as too sedated to be aware of their surroundings or happenings (Puntillo, 1994).

Clinical Pearl

A point to remember: Sedation is not analgesia. The use of sedative agents without an analgesic will leave the patient unable to communicate pain but still able to experience pain. A sedative agent such as propofol with an analgesic agent is a better combination to provide some element of pain relief. Additional analgesics may be needed after assessment with a BPS that indicates the presence of pain in a ventilated, sedated patient.

If the critically ill patient is restless and agitated, it may mean that he or she is experiencing pain. As always, it is prudent to provide an analgesic trial for the patient who has a condition that is known to be painful. Monitoring the effect of the analgesic can be measured by observing reduced levels of restlessness or agitation as compared with preanalgesia in a patient with unrelieved pain.

Monitoring the critically ill patient for the presence of pain is an important part of the plan of care. By assessing and providing pain medication for patients who are too ill to self-report pain, the patient will experience less stress and continue to discharge with a better physical and mental condition.

Procedural Pain Management

There are a large number of procedures performed in all the areas addressed in this chapter. Procedural pain has been an area that has been overlooked because most procedures are felt to be quick and relatively painless by those who are performing them. From the patient's perspective, however, procedural pain is something to be dreaded and the time seems to lag during the procedure.

In a study of pain related to procedures being performed in an ER, researchers questioned approximately 1,200 patients about the pain they experienced with their procedures. The patients ranked the most painful procedures as follows:

1. Nasogastric intubation
2. Abscess incision and drainage
3. Fracture reduction
4. Urinary catheter insertion (Singer, 1999)

The practitioners who performed the procedures ranked them in a similar fashion. When the two groups, patients and practitioners, were asked which procedures were less painful, the responses were ranked as follows:

1. IV insertion
2. Drawing blood gases
3. Local anesthesia
4. Lumbar puncture
5. Blood drawing
6. Suturing (Singer, 1999)

Of the group of 1,200 patients, only 12.8% had been offered analgesics prior to the procedure. The information from patients compared with the providers was highly variable when estimating pain. These findings indicate that it is critical to ask patients about pain when performing a procedure of any type and to offer analgesia (Singer, 1999).

In the critical care setting, a large multicenter study of 6,200 patients (Puntillo et al., 2001), which included both adults and children, studied the intensity of pain during several different types of procedures. The researchers asked the patients to rate the pain using a 0–100 pain scale for children and the 0–10 numeric rating scale (NRS) for adolescents and adults.

- For children, turning in bed was rated as 28–60 and tracheal suctioning was rated as 52–56 on the 100-point scale.
- For adolescents, reported pain of wound drain removal was rated as 5–7 on the NRS.
- For adults, it was reported that bed turning was most painful at an NRS rating of 4.93

It is obvious in this group that procedures caused significant pain. The distress ratings for procedures was also quite high: adolescents rated their distress at 4.83–6.0 and adults rated their distress at 1.89–3.47. The pain that these patients experienced was described as sharp, stinging, stabbing, shooting, and awful (Puntillo et al., 2001). Of note, less than 20% of all patients received opiates before any of the procedures (Puntillo et al., 2001).

In other research, a descriptive study of 31 surgical patients reported that pain was the most common sensation during drain removal, and they rated the pain at 4 on the NRS (Mimnaugh, Winegar, Mabrey, & Davis, 1999). In another descriptive study, 45 adult patients reported their pain at 7 on the NRS with endotracheal suctioning (Puntillo, 1994).

Based on patient reports, most of the procedures that are performed on patients are painful. However, most of the patients receive very little in the way of analgesics or local anesthetics. Recommendations for pain relief during procedures include:

- Make a regular pain assessment and reassessment.
- Use a BPS if the patient is nonverbal and note any recognized pain behaviors, such as grimacing, moaning, or increases in body tension.

- Use a topical anesthetic cream or a local intradermal anesthetic to decrease the pain associated with venipuncture.
- Use a lidocaine spray or combine it with a lidocaine jelly when inserting a nasogastric tube.
- Medicate the patient for pain or ensure that the patient receives an anesthetic agent before a procedure such as a bone marrow aspiration.
- Make sure the patient receives an analgesic before a procedure such as a chest tube removal.
- Use eutectic mixture of local anesthetic (EMLA) cream when performing wound care, as ordered, for at least 20 minutes before cleaning, debriding, or dressing the wound (D'Arcy, 2008).

In some cases, procedural sedation is needed to perform the procedure. This is a new area of practice, and hospitals have set up procedures and policies surrounding the practice that define who may provide this service and what types of medications can be used. Minimal and moderate sedation can be used. Moderate sedation is defined as patent airway and responsive to verbal commands or light tactile stimulation. Monitoring parameters are required with oxygen saturation, cardiac monitoring, and blood pressure measurements done throughout the sedation period (Todd & Miner, 2010). Patients who undergo mild, moderate, or even deep sedation may be amnesic about the events during the procedure. Common medications used for sedation are propofol (Diprivan), ketamine (Ketalar), etomidate (Amidate), and a combination of fentanyl (Sublimaze) and midazolam (Versed) (Todd & Miner, 2010).

For most patients who are undergoing a procedure, providing pain medication or some types of local anesthetic numbing medications will make the experience less painful and distressing. For other procedures, sedation at some level is required. Using complementary methods with analgesics can help the patient relax when the procedure is being performed. Providing pain relief during procedures is an important aspect of clinical care in critical care or ER settings.

Case Study

Jim Smith, 36 years old, was struck by a bus while crossing the street. He is being treated in the ER for multiple fractures, flail chest, and a closed head injury (a concussion). He is moaning and winces when he is moved or touched. He is asking for his wife and says he wants her to help him. Using a behavioral pain assessment tool, the nurse rates Jim's pain at 8/10. Jim has a pneumothorax that needs a chest tube, and it is placed without any analgesics. The respiratory status improves, but his heart rate increases, as does his blood pressure. The orthopedic team attempts to move his fractured leg and Jim screams out in pain. His wife asks if there isn't some way to provide pain relief for her husband who is obviously in pain.

Questions to Consider

1. Can we give Jim opioids? If so, what would you suggest?
2. Is Jim a candidate for an epidural for managing his flail chest pain? What would be the advantage of using an epidural?
3. Should they have medicated Jim before placing the chest tube?
4. What impact can the lack of adequate pain management have on the outcome of Jim's hospitalization?

REFERENCES

American College of Emergency Physicians. (2002). Critical issues in the evaluation of adult patients presenting to the emergency department with acute blunt abdominal trauma. Policy statement from the American College of Emergency Physicians. *Annals of Emergency Medicine, 43*(2), 278–290.

American Pain Society. (2008). *Principles of analgesic use in the treatment of acute pain and cancer pain*. Glenview, IL: The Society.

Blunt Thoracic Trauma Guideline. (2004). Retrieved from www.guideline.gov

Cordell, W. H., Keene, K. K., Giles, B. K., Jones, J. B., Jones, J. H., & Brizendine, E. J. (2002). The high prevalence of pain in emergency medical care. *American Journal of Emergency Medicine, 20*, 165–169.

D'Arcy, Y. (2008). Procedural pain alleviation. In B. Ackley, B. Swan, G. Ladwig, & S. Tucker (Eds.), *Evidence-based nursing care guidelines.* Philadelphia, PA: Mosby.

Erstad, B. L., Puntillo, K., Gilbert, H. C., Grap, M. J., Li, D., Medina, J., . . . Sessler, C. N. (2009). Pain management principles in the critically ill. *The Cardiopulmonary and Critical Care Journal, 135*(40), 1075–1086.

Horwitz, L. I., & Bradley, E. H. (2009). Percentage of US emergency department patients seen within the recommended triage time. *Archives of Internal Medicine, 169*(20), 1857–1865.

Jacobi, J., Fraser, G., Coursin, D., Riker, R., Fontaine, D., Wittbrodt, E., . . . Lumb, P. (2002). Clinical practice guidelines for the sustained use of sedatives and analgesics in the critically ill adult. *Critical Care Medicine, 30*(1), 1–42.

Mimnaugh, L., Winegar, M., Mabrey, Y., & Davis, J. E. (1999). Sensations experienced during removal of tubes in acute postoperative patients. *Applied Nursing Research, 12*(2), 78–85.

Mularski, R., Sessler, C., & Schmidt, G. (2010). Pain management in the intensive care unit. In *Bonica's management of pain* (4th ed.). Philadelphia, PA: Lippincott Williams & Wilkins.

Puntillo, K. (1994). Dimensions of procedural pain and its analgesic management in critically ill surgical patients. *American Journal of Critical Care, 3*(2), 116–122.

Puntillo, K., White, C., Morris, A., Perdue, S., Stanik-Hutt, J., Thompson, C., & Wild, L. (2001). Patients' perceptions and responses to procedural pain: Results form the Thunder Project II. *American Journal of Critical Care, 10*(4), 238–251.

Singer, A. J. (1999). Comparison of patients and practitioner assessments of pain from commonly performed emergency department procedures. *Annals of Emergency Medicine, 33*(6), 652–658.

Todd, K. (2010). Pain and prescription monitoring programs in the emergency department. *Annals of Emergency Medicine, 56*(1), 24–26.

Todd, K., Cowan, P., & Kelly, N. (in press). Chronic or recurrent pain in the emergency department: A national telephone survey of patient experience. *Western Journal of Emergency Medicine.*

Todd, K., & Miner, J. (2010). Pain management in the emergency department. In *Bonica's management of pain*. Philadelphia, PA: Lippincott Williams & Wilkins.

Index

Note: Page numbers followed by *f* indicate figures, *t* indicate tables, and *e* indicate exhibits.

O

P